THE ORIENTING REFLEX

PSYCHOLOGICAL STUDIES

MINOR SERIES 3

MOUTON · THE HAGUE · PARIS

THE ORIENTING REFLEX

E. H. VAN OLST

MOUTON - THE HAGUE - PARIS

Printed in the Netherlands.

The investigation as well as the present publication have been made possible through a grant from the Netherlands Organization for the Advancement of Pure Research (ZWO).

CONTENTS

PART II AN INVESTIGATION OF SOME PROPERTIES AND FUNCTIONS OF THE OR

INTRODUCTION

The phenomenon of the orienting reflex (OR), which was discovered by Pavlov as early as the beginning of this century, has not been extensively investigated until after 1945. At first, research was mainly confined to the Soviet Union, where, as is well known, Pavlov's ideas still dominate the psychological scene. Since 1960, western scientists have evinced a growing interest in Russian psychology, primarily focusing on the orienting reflex and related problems.

As for the place this subject occupies within psychology, the OR can be included under psychophysiology, which term should then not be taken in the old sense of sensory psychology and sensory physiology.

The domain of psychophysiology has recently (Stern, 1964) been defined as the study of the relations between psychological and physiological variables, the former being treated as independent, the latter as dependent variables. Consequently, such topics as classical conditioning, habituation and dishabituation, activation, etc are regarded as belonging to psychophysiology. The significance of psychophysiological research, while vital to functional psychology, is by no means confined to this field. From a methodological point of view, in particular, psychophysiology has proved its importance for clinical, social and developmental psychology, as well as for the study of individual differences as part of personality theory.

The influence of cognitive factors on the physiological substratum has increasingly found recognition in recent years. Thus, Sternbach (1964) concludes his article on the effect of the instructional variable on autonomic responsivity with the remark:

> 'It is no longer enough simply to have a subject stick his foot in ice water, or hear a bell, or look at a color slide, while we measure his heart rate, sweating, etc. We have shown that his physiological changes will be determined at least in part by what he thinks will happen, or by what the

> subject thinks *we* think will happen. This makes a difference, and it is an important one.'

In this study, some properties of the OR and some of their implications for experimental psychology will be investigated. Part I sets out the main hypotheses and investigations. Part II presents the results of our research.

PART I

PROPERTIES AND FUNCTIONS OF THE OR

1 THE PHENOMENON AND ITS DETERMINANTS

1.1 INTRODUCTION

In 1910 Pavlov discovered the orienting reflex, which in 1927 he described as follows: 'It is this reflex which brings about the immediate response in man and animal to the slightest changes in the world around them, so that they immediately orientate their appropriate receptor organ in accordance with the perceptible quality in the agent bringing about the change, making full investigation of it.'

Initially, only the immediately observable behavior components of this reaction were known, as for instance the turning of the head, pricking up of the ears, etc. The efforts of Russian investigators, in particular, have shown, however, that various changes occurring in the sense organs, in the autonomic and in the central nervous system as well as in the muscles should also be included in the OR pattern. Extensive reviews of these changes have been given by Sokolov (1963 b) and Berlyne (1960). Sokolov (1960) describes the OR as a non-specific reflex evoked by any (perceptible) stimulus change and extinguished through habituation upon repetition of the same stimulus change.

The main components of the reaction pattern are:

a) changes in the muscles, manifesting themselves in increased muscle tonus and receptor orientation.
b) increased sensory sensitivity (threshold lowering).
c) increased cortical arousal.
d) reactions in the autonomic nervous system, including decreased electrodermal resistance, vasoconstriction in the extremities, vasodilatation in the forehead, changes in respiration rate and heart rate.

The OR is closely related to the reticular activating system, which maintains a certain activation level of the cortical neurons. The activity of this system is determined not only by an internal rhythmicity (Oswald, 1962) but also by a not very specific sensory input. The latter may be considered the afferent mechanism of the OR. The efferent mechanism of the OR consists of somatic, sensory and autonomic components.

In the past, attention has been heavily concentrated on the effects of the reticular formation on the cortical processes (cortical arousal). Granit (1955), however, has demonstrated that the reticular system also plays a part in the regulation of receptor sensitivity. Reticular activation of the vasomotor system and the pupil (both are part of the efferent mechanism of the OR) has been demonstrated by Bonvallet, Dell and Hiebel (1954).

Dell (1963) found that direct stimulation of the reticular formation caused autonomic activity (autonomic arousal), manifesting itself in an electrodermal response. For a more detailed analysis of the arousal processes we refer to Van Olst and Orlebeke (1967).

1.2 DETERMINANTS OF THE OR

1.2.1 Novelty and change

The terms novelty, change, incongruity and the like are frequently used interchangeably. To arrive at a serviceable classification and description of the OR-determinants it is important to distinguish between the determinants which evoke the OR upon a first presentation of the stimulus, and the OR-determinants that are operative when after repeated presentations a change in stimulation is introduced. Properly speaking, the term 'novel' should only be used for the application of a first stimulus, that is, before any habituation has occurred. Novelty implies a high degree of uncertainty, which decreases upon repetition of the stimulus. The decrement is a sign of habituation. In the literature, however, we often find the term 'novelty' used with reference to a stimulus change. Sokolov (1966b) himself distinguishes two 'characteristics of novelty' based on the following two phenomena.

a) 'The reflex arising at the moment of application of the stimulus later disappears against the background of the continuing action of the stimulus; upon removal of the stimulus the reflex reappears.'
b) 'Arising upon the first appearance of the temporarily acting stimulus the reflex then weakens and completely disappears during repeated applications of the stimulus.'

These phenomena are not merely different aspects of the same process, since the effect mentioned under a) also occurs in decorticated animals, whereas in higher animals the occurrence mentioned under b) clearly requires some cortical mechanism. Whenever 'novelty' is used without further specification, it will refer to the process mentioned under b).

Sokolov (1966[b]) has shown that within a given stimulus sequence the degree of uncertainty at any single moment can in principle be determined by means of the Bayes theorem. The OR will occur if this uncertainty exceeds a certain value, which Sokolov calls the 'threshold of novelty'. Modification of the stimulus after a number of repetitions can in principle be regarded as the introduction of a new stimulus. If the modified stimulus is in any respect in conflict with the (perceptual) expectation of the observer, we prefer to use the term 'incongruity'. Alternatively, the term can be used in a negative sense, when an expected change fails to occur.

There are good grounds for introducing the concept of incongruity. Stimulus change (the occurrence of a new stimulus) in itself does not necessarily evoke an OR. The change will frequently involve physical properties (and their sensory correlates), but only certain dimensions will be relevant to the observer. If the stimulus change is at variance with the (experimentally) induced expectation, one will speak of incongruity, which in principle corresponds to the distinction drawn by Prokasy and Hall (1963) between events as seen by the experimenter, and as they appear to the subject. When very elementary stimuli (*e.g.* pure tones) are used, stimulus change and incongruity may coincide. The ability to react to the factor 'change' (incongruity) presupposes at least a detection mechanism capable of checking afferent signals against some kind of memory in which information about previous stimuli is stored for a certain length of time. Any incongruity between input and memory would evoke an OR. Sokolov (1960) has suggested such a mechanism under the name of 'neuronal model of the stimulus', which will be discussed in due course.

Following Sokolov, many authors have investigated the OR-evoking character of stimulus changes (Berlyne, 1960; Berlyne, Craw, Salapatek and Lewis, 1963; Williams, 1963; Allen, Hill and Wickens, 1963; Hayes, Bronsaft, Bloch and Welch, 1964). These investigations confirmed Sokolov's view that stimulus change is OR-evoking.

Contrariwise, Fried, Korn and Welch (1966) arrived at the conclusion that 'novelty is not a fact, but a dimension which is not presently understood'.

Their experimental design was based on the presentation of a series of stimuli without inter-stimulus intervals. Four circular colored stimuli (green, blue, white or amber) were presented in apparent random order, each for 7.5 sec. The entire series consisted of 80 stimuli, all colors occurring with equal frequency. When the 11th amber stimulus was due, the experimental group received a red stimulus. For the experimental as well as for the control group, each consisting of 20 subjects, curves were drawn up for the amber stimulus (20 trials), showing the absolute electrodermal resistance as plotted against the serial numbers of the stimulus presentations. There proved to be no significant difference between the two groups, so that the authors concluded that the novelty of the (red) stimulus apparently has no effect, *i.e.* does not evoke an OR.

With a minor variation this investigation was repeated by Fried, Welch, Friedman and Gluck (1967), who left out either the 6th, the 11th, or the 16th amber stimulus. Neither the position of a stimulus in the sequence, nor its elimination was found to produce any effect. The design and execution of these investigations, however, do not warrant the authors' interpretation that their results refute the existence of a 'novelty' factor as intended by Sokolov, since the latter defines the OR as a phasic change in, among other things, electrodermal conductance, whereas Fried and his co-authors regard a tonic change (the absolute dermal resistance) as the response category. Moreover, Sokolov (1966[b]) uses the term 'novelty' as referring to discrete stimulations with distinct inter-stimulus intervals. It is not unlikely that, because of the absence of any intertrial stimulus intervals, no expectations as to sequence are aroused in a serial procedure as adopted by Fried and his associates.

The measuring techniques employed by these authors have been sharply criticized by Furedy (1968, 1969), who, in a comparative investigation of the various response categories, found phasic changes in electrodermal conductance to be the best measure for determining the influence of stimulus changes. Absolute electrodermal resistance was found to show little or no differentiation with respect to the new stimulus. Consequently, Furedy attributes the negative results obtained by Fried *et al.* to inappropriate methods of measurement.

Berlyne (1961, 1968), and Weiner and Feltman (1967) have treated the concept of novelty in terms of information theory. Berlyne (1961) found that for complex stimuli (words) with a high information value the OR was significantly stronger than for word stimuli with a low information value ($p < .01$).

The information value of the stimulus words employed had been determined by Laffal (quoted by Berlyne) on the basis of the number of associations evoked. Upon hearing a stimulus word, subjects in Berlyne's experiment had to name the first association that came to mind. In a later investigation (Berlyne *et al.*, 1968), Berlyne formulated the hypothesis that subjective uncertainty caused by blurred pictures will intensify the OR. This situation is to be considered a form of conflict or competition between response tendencies corresponding to alternative hypotheses. Blurred pictures proved to cause more prolonged blocking of the alpha-rhythm than did clear pictures. In the GSR, however, no difference was found.

The alpha-blocking did not occur when just before the presentation of the blurred picture, the clear picture had been presented.

Like Berlyne, Weiner and Feltman (1967) start from the assumption that the amount of information contained in a stimulus depends, among other things, on its 'novelty'. They go on to state that the amount of information that can be processed per time-unit is determined by the channel capacity.

An experiment was carried out to test the hypothesis that when during an auditory signal-detection task (vigilance experiment) a visual stimulus is introduced as noise, detection is impaired to an extent that will decrease with increasing exposure time of the visual stimulus. At first the new visual stimulus will take up part of the channel capacity, but with increasing exposure time the information value of the visual stimulus will diminish as its 'novelty' decreases. Experimental confirmation of the hypothesis was obtained. In this experiment the OR played an important part. The new (visual) stimulus evokes an OR which is stronger if the information value of the stimulus is higher, or in other words, if the stimulus is more 'novel'. This OR causes inhibition of the 'ongoing behavior', in this case the signal-detection task (cp Ch 2.1). In the course of the stimulus presentation the OR-effect disappears at the same rate as the information value decreases.

1.2.2 Conflict and surprise

When in discrimination learning the positive and the negative stimuli show great similarity, an intermediate stimulus will evoke a strong OR. According to Pavlov, a conflict situation is involved which is strongly OR-evocative. Even without perceptual discrimination difficulties, conflict evokes an OR, as was demonstrated by Berlyne (1961), who realized low-conflict and high-conflict trials by means of 'free choice' and 'forced choice' situations. The stimulus situation was as follows: 'For low-conflict trials, two lights at one corner of the diamond were illuminated whereas, for high-conflict trials, two lights at different corners were illuminated.'

A stimulus series consisted of 12 low-conflict trials and 12 high-conflict trials, distributed at random. The subjects were instructed to press down a key capable of moving in four directions, corresponding to the four corners of the diamond. The low-conflict trials consisted of a forced choice situation in which the key was to be moved in the direction of the two lights. The high-conflict trials, on the other hand, entailed a free choice situation: the key could be moved in either direction, depending on the subject's choice.

To achieve optimal isolation of the 'conflict' factor, the stimulus was presented for 10 seconds, the subjects being required to react upon disappearance of the stimulus. When the OR's occurring at the onset of the stimulus were studied, it was found that those belonging to the high-conflict trials were significantly larger than those occurring in the low-conflict trials ($p < .01$).

Berlyne (1961) has also attempted to isolate the 'surprise' factor. According to him, 'surprise' is a specific form of the conflict situation. On the one hand, a response tendency exists on the basis of a certain expectation; on the other hand, a stimulus which is at variance with the expectation will induce a response incompatible with the earlier response. A series of stimuli incorporating the surprise factor but without novelty of the stimuli was obtained in the following way. Two visual stimuli of equal intensity were presented, consisting of two lights, A and B, in the order ABABAB etc.. By way of surprise, the 16th stimulus substituted A for B, after which the sequence was continued normally, BAA being followed by the regular ABAB. The substitution had not been announced. The 19th stimulus, again an A, served as control stimulus. A second sequence was announced as BABA etc. In this series, the 19th stimulus, a B, was changed to A (surprise stimulus), the 16th stimulus, again an A, serving as control. The difference between the OR's, measured as the difference in GSR between the surprise and control stimuli, was highly significant ($p < .001$).

1.2.3 Intensity

Both Sokolov (1963[b]) and Asafov (1958) have found a J-type correlation between the magnitude of the OR and the stimulus intensity. According to Asafov, this effect – an initial decrease of the OR with increasing stimulus intensity (reckoned from the absolute threshold) followed by a continuous increase – is the result of two separate processes. In his view, stimulus values close to the absolute threshold can be perceived only as 'present' or 'not present'. When now the stimulus intensity is gradually stepped up, the differences between the successive stimuli will initially be so slight that the stimuli are perceived as identical, with the result that the OR is to some extent extinguished. Once sufficiently strong stimuli cause the intensity as such to dominate, the OR magnitude becomes a linear function of the intensity.

According to Sokolov, the curve for auditory stimuli shows an upward trend around 50 db.

Leavy and Geer (1967) repeated this experiment and analyzed the results rigorously. Four groups, each consisting of 12 persons, received stimuli of 20, 30, 40, or 50 db respectively. Unlike Sokolov, they found a positive linear function for the entire range. For another part of the scale, from 70 to 120 db, similar outcomes were obtained by Davis, Buchwald and Frankmann (1955), whose results were in accordance with the findings of Hovland and Riessen (1940). This linear relation was found to exist not only for tone stimuli but for white noise as well. With respect to the latter, Uno and Grings (1965) found a linear relation for the 60–100 db range at 10 db intervals.

1.2.4 Perceptual expectation

In many cases, the occurrence of an OR can be considered the result of a discrepancy between the perceptual expectation and the actual event. Postman and Bruner (quoted by Bruner, 1951) describe perception in terms of a 'hypothesis-information-confirmation cycle', its three phases comprising:

1. the formation – on the basis of previous occurrences – of a certain expectation or hypothesis
2. intake of information
3. a confirmation process, in which the information is found to be either congruent or incongruent with the hypothesis or expectation.

With regard to the strength of the hypothesis Bruner formulated three postulates:

1. the stronger the hypothesis, the more likely it is to be aroused
2. the stronger the hypothesis, the less information will be needed for its confirmation
3. the stronger the hypothesis, the more information will be needed for its negation.

The strength of the hypothesis is, in a positive sense, determined by the following factors:

a) the number of previous confirmations	frequency principle
b) the number of alternatives	monopoly principle
c) its plausibility, *i.e.* the number of other hypotheses supporting it	cognitive factor
d) the extent to which certain goals can be realized after confirmation of the hypothesis	motivation factor
e) the degree of correspondence with hypotheses of other observers.	social factor

In any case, the strength of a hypothesis is not a simple linear function of the frequency of its occurrence: the effect of an unexpected event is greatest on the first presentation. After this first presentation, the threshold will be considerably lowered, or in other words, the chance that from the observer's point of view a certain event will take place will increase greatly. Instructional variables, in particular, exercise a strong influence. It is important, therefore, to distinguish between the relevancy to the experimenter of the information provided, and the observer's interpretation of this information. The observer has his own notions about the probability of certain events manifesting themselves.

A good illustration is the influence of affective factors. The probability of stimuli with positive significance occurring is generally overestimated, that of stimuli with a negative significance underestimated. In a probability learning experiment Rosenhan and Messick (1966) used as stimuli angry and laughing faces and small and big kangaroos, the latter as control stimuli. In certain series laughing faces and big kangaroos made up 70% of the total series as against 30% in others; each series consisted of 150 stimuli. In the series containing 70% angry faces the occurrence of negative stimuli was underestimated (average estimate 57.5%). In the series containing 70% laughing faces, the estimates (average 68.2) did not deviate much from objective probability.

In the two kangaroo series the percentages were 63.8 and 65.8. Individual differences proved considerable in the series containing affective stimuli. The differences were partly related to personality differences (determined by means of Edwards' Personal Preference Schedule).

Solley and Murphy (1960) have likewise stressed the role of the expectation factor in perception: 'Perceptual expectation is the first molar unit of the perceptual act, a unit which continues at least until the percept is achieved.'

The second phase in perception is that of attention, which is partly determined by the first phase. In the third phase, that of reception, the sensory input begins to play a role. Between receipt of stimulation and the ultimate percept there is yet another phase, which Solley and Murphy designate as 'trial and check': 'In this molar unit hypotheses are tested, unconscious assumptions are checked and materials supplied by the sensory process are articulated with previously stored memoric traces.' This phase corresponds to Bruner's 'confirmation procedure'.

Simultaneously with this trial and check process, and interacting with it, there occurs a process of arousal. (The OR in the form of arousal response can be regarded as an aspect of the arousal process – see Van Olst and Orlebeke, 1967). Solley and Murphy assign the onset of an OR to the second phase, that of attention. In the case of a first, new stimulus, this is undoubtedly correct. However, an OR will likewise occur whenever in the 'trial and check' phase expectation and receipt of stimulation prove to be incongruent.

Grings (1960) calls this the 'perceptual disparity response', of which he says: 'It is defined as the difference in magnitude of response between situations where receipt of stimulation following a signal cue is in accord with past experience and where receipt of stimulation is not in accord with past experience with the particular cue.' Or to put it differently, the OR permits investigation of the occurrence and development of certain expectancy patterns. Solley and Murphy's remark that there are 'no independent measures of expectancy and perception' therefore does not appear to be quite correct.

1.2.5 Signal Value

In Russian psychology it is usual to divide stimuli into two main categories, signal and non-signal stimuli. Stimuli without signal value are classified as neutral and of no specific significance to the observer. Sokolov (1963[b]), following Anokhin, defines signal stimuli as 'stimuli which evoke a reaction in anticipation of external agents likely to appear in the future'. He regards as particularly significant 'the acquired features of the stimuli which are the signals for certain reactions'. In general, a neutral stimulus can acquire signal value in three different ways (Lynn, 1966):

1. Through classical conditioning, in which a neutral stimulus is transformed into a conditional stimulus, which acts as a signal for the occurrence of the non-conditional stimulus

2. By instructing the subject to perform a certain action at the onset of the stimulus
3. By instructing the subject to pay attention to a certain stimulus.

The process whereby signal value is acquired can be designated as signalization. Significantly, the conditioning process is thereby placed within a wider framework. It may be added that the first method of signalization occurs in the so-called first signal system, while the second method forms, as it were, the transition to the so-called second signal system, by which Pavlov designated the verbal system. Now, the OR which is evoked by signal stimuli is stronger and continues much longer than in the case of non-signal stimuli. This is seen quite clearly when the subject hears his own name pronounced.

The importance of the third signalization method – attention focusing through verbal instruction – has recently been demonstrated by Korn and Moyer (1968). Two groups with different experimental conditions received a series of tones. The first group had been instructed to relax and pay no special attention to the tones. The second group were likewise told to relax, but they were given the additional instruction: 'Stay alert and pay attention to the tones you will hear. Be ready for whatever might happen.' The OR's of the two groups differed significantly.

1.2.6 Other cognitive factors

In the preceding pages cognitive aspects of the determinants involved in the modification of stimuli have been discussed. In order is now a discussion of the cognitive stimulus characteristics that determine the OR when the stimulus is first presented. Berlyne and his associates have investigated the relation between the OR and what they call 'collative properties of stimulus patterns'. By this they understand such attributes as novelty, surprise, complexity and incompatibility. The factors 'novelty' and 'surprise' have already been dealt with, so we shall confine our attention to the last two.

Complexity and incompatibility in the stimulus materials have been investigated by Berlyne, Craw, Salapatek and Lewis (1963). They used eight categories of visual stimuli, each category consisting of two pairs of patterns. Each pair was made up of a regular and an irregular pattern, the nature of the difference within each pair varying for all eight categories. The 16 pairs made up a total of 32 stimuli. There were four low-complexity categories and four high-complexity ones. Complexity related to the number of details in the figures used.

The four low-complexity categories concerned irregularity of arrangement, difference in amount of material, heterogeneity of the elements and irregularity of the shapes. These differences within the stimulus pairs were realized in simple geometrical figures.

The high-complexity categories (or at least three out of four) were based on the same principles, but the figures were composed of far more elements. Each stimulus pair of these more complex figures differed in respect of symmetry, randomization of the relative positions of the elements or the number of elements involved. The fourth category, that of incompatibility, will be discussed later.

Two experimental conditions were run: with and without extrinsic motivation. The former condition was realized by an instructional set requiring the subjects to pay close attention to the stimuli in preparation for a recognition test. Each stimulus was presented three times, for 3 sec, with an interstimulus interval of 12 sec. The response measure was the GSR calculated as $\triangle$ log C. There were 80 subjects. The series were arranged in such a manner as to eliminate all kinds of sequence effects.

Extrinsic motivation was found to have a significant effect on the number of GSR's (p. $< .001$). In the group without induced motivation no differences were found, either between regular and irregular patterns or between low and high complexity. In the extrinsically motivated group, on the other hand, the difference between regular and irregular patterns proved significant (p. $< .026$), but not that between low and high complexity. The conclusion is that with extrinsic motivation irregular patterns evoke more GSR's.

As a special case of the factor 'irregularity' in complex patterns, a form of conflict or incompatibility was introduced, in the material itself. This intrinsic incompatibility was realized, for instance, in a birdlike shape with the hindquarters of a mammal. This type of 'irregularity' was found to produce a significant difference: for the two experimental conditions the p values were $p < .01$ and $p < .05$ respectively.

In a supplementary experiment the authors demonstrated that in the case of induced motivation there is a significant difference between the low-complexity and high-complexity groups ($p < .05$). Summation across the groups with and without motivation also produced a significant result ($p = .03$). The observed differences were all in the predicted direction, that is, more irregularity, greater complexity and induced motivation produced higher GSR values. This result was regarded as due to the greater information value of stimuli of this kind.

The importance of the attention variable of the OR was clearly brought out in this study.

1.2.7 Memory capacity

The subject matter of this section as well as the next relates to habituation of the OR. The habituation process itself will be dealt with in chapter 3.

Stern (1968) has attempted to relate various aspects of the OR to different memory forms. He thinks it likely that the OR decrement (habituation) which occurs when the stimulus is repeated is indicative of the short-term memory imprinting process. Short-term memory retention decreases as a function of time.This is held to find expression in the more rapid habituation occurring with shorter interstimulus intervals.

In addition, there is the so-called intersession habituation, which manifests itself in a decrease of the first response to a stimulus sequence repeated at long intervals (days or weeks). Stern regards this habituation as related to the long-term memory imprinting process. Accordingly, it is to be expected that long-term memory parameters will correlate highly with those of intersession habituation. To date no research on this subject has been published.

A lesser-known fact is that an OR occurs likewise upon termination of a relatively prolonged stimulus (Sokolov 1960). This observation has been confirmed by Stern. Habituation of these 'terminal' OR's is more rapid than habituation of 'onset' OR's.

A remarkable aspect is that terminal OR's occur much more massively (with greater frequency and regularity) at an early age. Thus Stern found that while there was no difference between six-year olds and twelve-year olds in speed of habituation for onset OR's, a difference did exist with regard to terminal OR's. In six-year olds habituation took three times as long. Stimulus change produced greater OR's in children than in adults; and these were even more pronounced in the case of terminal OR's.

As stated before, habituation of the onset OR can be interpreted as a decrease of the information value of the stimulus. Stern points out the connection between habituation of the terminal OR and the attention span, which he defines as the 'time binding ability of the organism'.

If the organism can conceptualize the duration of a stimulus, the terminal OR, if occurring, habituates quickly.

With regard to the two basic attributes, duration and content of the stimulus, the terminal OR is inversely proportional to the organism's ability to conceive or apprehend time, whereas the onset OR is related to the content of the stimulus.

Since apprehension of time in terms of duration is connected with attention span, and since the latter increases as a function of age and experience, it may be posited that measures of the attention span will show high negative correlations with the habituation rate of the terminal OR's. So far, however, developmental psychology has not made any headway with this type of research.

1.2.8 Individual differences

Although individual differences are borderline territory between experimental psychology and typology, they should be briefly mentioned here, since they constitute one of the OR determinants.

Roessler *et al.* (1963) and Greenfield *et al.* (1963) found that higher scores on the Barron ego strength scale of M.M.P.I. correlated positively with stronger GSR's and digital vasomotor reactions, measured as responses to standard tones. This held not only for the response amplitude, but also for the response duration.

Luborsky (1967) established that the magnitude of the OR to novel stimuli was in part determined by the 'individual's typical cognitive controls'. For each of twelve individuals he determined the mean of 10 vasomotor responses to a tone of 500 cps, 60 db, and calculated the rank correlation coefficient between these mean figures and the following variables:

Number of Rorschach responses	rho = .76
RT embedded figures	rho = —.64
Amount of deviation from the vertical in the rod and frame test	rho = —.46

The conclusion drawn from this is that the OR correlates positively with the individual's intake of information, that is, with his ability (or preference) to distinguish between stimulus and background.

Koepke and Pribram (1966) divided 40 subjects into two groups on the basis of their spontaneous activity, the criterion being the number of spontaneous GSR's > 1 K Ohm during the two minutes preceding the first stimulus presentation. All subjects whose spontaneous activity was below the median value were qualified as 'stable', the other subjects as 'unstable'.

The average habituation rate of the two groups was found to differ significantly (for the 'stable' group 5.5 trials, for the 'unstable' group 10.0 trials; $p < .02$).

The 'unstable' group were also found to have a shorter latency time ($p < .05$). The condition of 'stable' or 'unstable' had no effect on the response amplitude.

For each subject the score on the Taylor Anxiety scale was determined and correlated with the following variables:

Habituation rate	$r = .23$ (n.s.)
First response amplitude	$r = .16$ (n.s.)
Spontaneous activity	$r = .28$ ($p < 0.5$)

The same authors (Koepke and Pribram, 1967) conducted a similar experiment in which vasoconstriction in the fingers served as the dependent variable. Here the correlation between the subjects' T.A.S. scores and their habituation rate was found to be much higher ($r = .51$: $p < .01$).

1.2.9 Social factors

Finally, it should be pointed out that in all likelihood social-psychological factors, and in particular small-group social interaction, also affect the OR. Research in this area has been conducted by, among others, Kaplan, Burch and Bloom (1965), Shapiro and Leiderman (1965), Nowling, Eisdorfer Bogdonoff and Nichols (1968) and Costell and Leiderman (1968). It would take us too far afield to go into details.

2 FUNCTIONS OF THE OR

2.1 GENERAL FUNCTIONS

One of the most important functions of the OR is adjustment of the analyzers. By analyzer we understand the whole of receptor, projection system, the specific cortical area and the efferent system which provides feedback to the analyzer (Sokolov, 1967). Each analyzer consists of a combination of different afferent systems (Sokolov, 1963[b]). Thus the 'skin analyzer' comprises the senses of pain, pressure, warmth and cold. Even a single stimulation of this analyzer will elicit a complex of temporally differentiated phenomena which as such reach the neuronal center. One of the reasons for this is that the thresholds and rates of impulse transmission differ in the various afferent systems.

It is important to distinguish the OR from another type of regulation in the analyzer, *viz.* adaptation. A characteristic difference between orienting and adaptive reflexes is, among other things, the occurrence, after habituation of an initial OR, of a new OR as a result of a slight stimulus change, whereas no adaptive reflexes occur. Another difference concerns the nature of the stimulation. Unlike the OR, adaptive reflexes are evoked only by adequate (specific) stimuli. If the stimulus intensity exceeds a certain value and the adaptive reflexes can no longer provide adequate regulation, defensive reflexes will occur. Both adaptive and defensive reflexes serve to restrict the effect of the stimulus, the operation of an adaptive reflex being limited to a specific analyzer, whereas defensive reflexes extend to the entire organism.

This last qualification also applies to the OR, but the latter reinforces the stimulus effect. In general, the OR precedes the adaptive reflexes, but where defensive reflexes are concerned, the stimulus intensity is the determining factor. According to Sokolov (1963[b]), a weak pain stimulus will evoke an OR, but repeated stimulation will elicit a defensive reflex. Strong pain stimuli immediately evoke a defensive reflex. Compared to the OR, the defensive reflex habituates very slowly if at all. Within the intensity dimension we can thus distinguish a certain range of stimulus values which upon first presentation evoke only an OR. This range is extended downwards as well as upwards as soon as the stimuli acquire signal value.

Sokolov (1960, 1963[b]) further differentiates between the tonic and phasic forms of the OR and between generalized and localized orientation reflexes. The tonic form manifests itself in the maintenance for some considerable time of a certain level of activation or arousal, whereas the phasic form represents a rapid and brief activation or increase of arousal, elicited by a single stimulus.

Initially, the OR occurs in all the analyzers as a generalized reflex, but with stimulus repetition the OR gradually becomes confined to the analyzer of the specific stimulus modality – the localized OR.

The occurrence of an OR frequently causes inhibition of the ongoing behavior. In this connexion Anokhin (1965) has formulated the so-called exclusion principle: 'Every holistic activity of the organism has a tendency to be the only one present at a given time and to exclude all other acts. The organism cannot combine simultaneously two or three holistic activities'.

The interactions which according to Anokhin may attend the occurrence of an OR are threefold:

a) *conflict*

By virtue of the exclusion principle, and depending on the intensity of the excitation process, many other activities are inhibited.

b) *assimilation*

The OR is assimilated by the organism's ongoing activity and contributes to the dominant condition preceding it. This means that the OR excitation is summated with the organism's temporally dominating activity. An instance of this would be the reinforcement of a defensive reflex by a new stimulus.

c) *transformation*

Under the influence of an OR, a latent 'dominanta' becomes manifest (What Anokhin means by the term 'dominanta' is not quite clear; probably, hierarchically related behavioral units are intended). This can be demonstrated by the following example: If an animal, in a situation in which it is accustomed to receive food, is presented with a new stimulus, assimilation with the pre-existing food 'dominanta' will occur. If, however, in the same situation an unpleasant electrical shock had been applied some considerable time before, a new stimulus will primarily elicit the defensive dominanta instead of the food dominanta. In the latter case the OR has undergone transformation.

The conclusion may be drawn that the general OR pattern is not isolated from the rest of the organism's behavior. Whenever an OR occurs, one of the above interactions is involved.

2.2 THE FUNCTION OF THE OR IN THE CONDITIONING PROCESS

Although it has become quite apparent that the OR plays an important part in the majority of behavioral processes, this field is still almost entirely unexplored, except for the function of the OR in classical conditioning, about which a good deal is known.

2.2.1 Introduction

By classical conditioning we understand (Thorpe, 1956): 'the process of acquisition by an animal of the capacity to respond to a given stimulus with the reflex reaction proper to another stimulus (the reinforcement) when the two stimuli are applied concurrently for a number of times'. This definition we regard as applicable also to man.

In practice, the conditioning of motor reactions in man is far from easy as well as time-consuming. For this reason autonomic responses forming part of a defensive reaction have often been used for conditioning. This approach tacitly assumes that the conditioning of autonomic responses can be subsumed under the classical conditioning model. Historically, however, this model has been developed from results obtained in the conditioning of motor reactions and the salivary reflex. The question as to whether generalization of this model to autonomic conditioning is justified ties in closely with the issue of what role the OR plays in the conditioning process. Before we attempt to deal with this problem, a few words must be said about the conditioning model itself.

2.2.2 Assumptions and concepts

Classical conditioning is predicated on the reflex concept, that is, it requires the existence of a stimulus-response relation falling within the reflex category.

Repeated presentations of the UCS (unconditional stimulus) must continue to evoke a measurable UCR (unconditioned response).

The second condition is that the CS (conditional stimulus) for the acquisition procedure must not elicit the UCR, or, in other words, must be neutral with respect to the UCR. Thirdly, during acquisition a CR (conditioned response) resembling the UCR must be established. No matter what UCS is chosen for defensive conditioning, it should always be borne in mind that in the case of a defensive reflex there is never a single response but rather a complex of responses.

Dykman (1967), who defines psychophysiology as 'the study of changes that occur in *multiple* end organs in the presence of some kind of stimulation or uniform background', therefore advocates a much more inclusive approach in conditioning studies. If only one response system is studied, all kinds of relations, such as the effect of respiration on other systems and individual differences in response pattern, will be overlooked.

A complication is caused by the fact that the CS itself elicits a response that used to be called alpha response in American publications and which is termed OR in the Russian literature. The usual practice is to have subjects, prior to the acquisition procedure, habituate this response. The presentation of the UCS during acquisition, however, causes sensitization, as a result of which the alpha response reappears. In terms of the Russian literature this means that the new stimulus combination evokes an OR, and, more specifically, an OR which is now determined by the signal value of the CS (signalization). For, after the first presentation of the CS-UCS combination, the CS will have come to signal the occurrence of the UCS. This signalization is apparent from the reoccurrence of the OR to the CS in the second CS-UCS combination.

The sensitization effect is sometimes termed pseudo-conditioning. These two notions, however, are not identical. In our view the phenomenon of a response resembling the UCR being evoked by the CS to a number of separate UCS presentations prior to presentation of the CS-UCS combination, should not, as Gormezano (1966) does, be called pseudo-conditioning, but simply sensitization. Sensitization can be equated with pseudo-conditioning only if the augmentation of the original response to the CS is due to a conditioning procedure. Dykman (1967) makes this observation on the relation between conditioning and pseudo-conditioning: 'True CR's reflect a plasticity function of the nervous system, pseudo-conditioned responses (PCR's) reflect some transitory change in threshold.'

Wickens and Wickens (1942) refer to CR's as 'associative modifications' and to PCR's as 'non-associative modifications'. These modifications or components are difficult to discriminate, the distinction being related to the difference between 'performance' and 'learning'. 'Performance' is an empirical fact, relating as it does to measurable behavioral responses, 'learning' is a theoretical notion whose existence is inferred from changes in 'performance' brought about by training or conditioning (Dykman, 1967).

Dykman arrives at this conclusion: 'All changes in performance occurring to the CS and prior to the UCS, or during the normal period of the UCS when it is omitted, whether the directional change is augmentation or habituation, result via one primary mechanism, sensitization.' Sensitization is defined by him as 'an increase of neural pathways either inhibitory or excitatory'. 'Learning', in his view, is a sensitization process 'in which pathways repeatedly used are altered'. Habituation of the sensitized response is thus to be regarded as part of the learning process.

2.2.3 The significance of the OR *for conditioning*

In principle Dykman's views tend in the same direction as Sokolov's. Sokolov (1963[b]) attributes to the OR an indispensable role in the conditioning process, which according to him is apparent from the dishabituation of the initially habituated OR to a CS at the start of the conditioning process. Owing to the occurrence of the OR the excitation level in the cortical centers is raised, both with respect to the CS and the UCS, which is conducive to establishing the relation between CS and UCS. During conditioning a kind of concentration of excitation takes place concomitantly with habituation of the OR to the CS. Sokolov (1960) states that at the start of the conditioning process stimulus generalization takes place, within the stimulus modality to which the CS belongs.

In the instance cited by him an auditory CS of 500 cps was applied, and it was found that initially stimuli in the 300–900 cps range likewise elicited the UCR (defensive reflex). In the course of the acquisition procedure this range diminished to 450–500 cps. So long as the CR has not been fully established and the OR to the CS is not yet habituated, there exists a relationship between the two responses which Lynn (1966) has termed 'reciprocal inhibition'. The OR inhibits the CR to give the organism time to evaluate the stimulus.

In any event, reciprocal inhibition plays a vital part in voluntary motor conditioning (VMC). In this process the UCS is a verbal instruction and the UCR a certain form of motor behavior. In the simplest form of the procedure the subject is given the instruction (UCS), on hearing a certain signal (CS), to press a key (UCR). The strength of the CR set in train (electrical activity in the muscles involved) can be established from the EMG and is inversely proportional to the degree of habituation of the OR. In other words, the CS initially evokes strong OR's but as yet no CR, while in the course of the conditioning process the OR is found to decrease and the CR to become established. This phenomenon can be regarded as a form of reciprocal inhibition (Sokolov, 1963[b]).

These facts raise the question whether the common practice of habituating the OR to the CS prior to the conditioning procedure is meaningful. It would rather seem that in fact an adverse effect must be produced. Sokolov (1963[b]) found that without previous habituation of the OR to the CS a VMC became established after 2 or 3 trials whereas 15 to 50 trials were required to achieve the same result if the OR to the CS was previously habituated. In this connection Sokolov quotes Konorsky and Shĕikovskaya, who demonstrated that if a particular stimulus had previously been used in a conditioning procedure, conditioning was much more difficult to establish. The renewed occurrence of the OR during conditioning depends on the subject's perceiving the relation 'if CS than UCS'. It is generally true that if the action proceeds completely automatically (optimal learning result), no OR develops.

The conclusion appears justified that the OR plays an essential part in the learning process. Luria (1963) points out that in mentally deficient subjects defects in attention and poor learning are due to defects in the OR mechanism and the habituation system. As a result, verbal behavior regulation can develop only imperfectly or not at all.

With regard to the testing phase in the conditioning process there is another point which deserves closer attention. The experimenter, when verifying whether a CR has in fact been established, will omit the UCS on the assumption that the CS will elicit the CR if present. However, omission of the UCS implies a novel stimulus situation. The consequences are twofold. First, an OR will be evoked and, secondly, the occurrence of this OR will to a greater or less extent inhibit the CR. If the experimenter at the same time verifies whether simulus generalization is taking place, there will be a third consequence: any stimuli other than the CS will likewise evoke an OR. Thus a simple change in procedure, *viz.* from acquisition to testing phase, already has far-reaching consequences. This last point, *viz.* the effect of introducing a test stimulus, has been clearly brought out in a study by Zimny and Kienstra (1967) on GSR conditioning.

Another important question concerns the conditioning criterion. What level should the CR attain in the acquisition period? Thompson (1965) reports an experimental study in which it was found that at an acquisition level of 50% there was still cross-modal generalization, but not at the 90% level. In the early stages of conditioning the organism still responds to a wide range of stimuli of different modalities. In the course of acquisition this range becomes progressively narrower until only stimuli of the same modality as the CS are generalized. This uni-modal range, in turn, narrows until a 100% acquisition level has been reached; put another way, the generalization gradient then attains its maximal slope. It follows that the criterion for acquisition must be set at 100% to permit an unambiguous appraisal of stimulus relations.

The question now is what is to be understood by this 100%. If the criterion is interpreted in the sense that the amplitude of the CR must be equal to that of the UCR, this method will as a rule be unfeasible. If one sets the criterion that the CR must, in a manner further to be stipulated, approach to a particular limit, it is most likely that for instance GSR conditioning cannot meet the requirement.

It is almost certain that in the early stages of conditioning the cortical association areas play a special role. According to Thompson, non-specific responses occurring in these early stages are associated with attention behavior. The extent of cortical activation, measured by means of the EEG, decreases progressively as conditioning advances. Presumably, this phenomenon is the same as the transition from the generalized to the localized OR, as described by Sokolov. Applications of the conditioning model are thus fraught with complications, at least as far as autonomic conditioning is concerned, which renders its practical utility smaller than is frequently assumed.

3 HABITUATION OF THE OR

3.1 INTRODUCTION

In the preceding pages the term habituation has repeatedly been used to denote the response decrement of the various OR components due to stimulus repetition. To some extent habituation may be regarded as the major characteristic of the OR as far as the continuity of behavior is concerned. In view of the importance of the habituation process a separate chapter will be devoted to it.

A generally accepted definition of the habituation phenomenon is that given by Harris (1943) as 'response decrement as a result of repeated stimulation'. This does not include the peripherally determined response decrement taking place in the receptors and effectors which Thompson and Spencer (1966) call 'receptor adaptation' and 'effector fatigue' respectively. In a sense, habituation may be regarded as a form of learning. It is difficult, however, to give a general definition of learning which is not so vague as to be almost meaningless. In any event, habituation manifests itself as a decrease of response intensity, and the same cannot be said of most learning processes.

Deese (1958), who unreservedly includes habituation in the learning process, gives this definition: 'Habituation is learning not to respond to stimuli which tend to be without significance in the life of the animal.' He elaborates this definition as follows: 'Habituation must be regarded as the most fundamental and elementary example of the permanent modification of behavior by repeated stimulation.'

3.2 PARAMETRIC CHARACTERISTICS

From the literature Thompson and Spencer (1966) have compiled a list of parametric characteristics, which is reproduced below. As the list was found to be incomplete, we have inserted additions in the appropriate places. Since the GSR is the most sensitive component of the OR and the present study will focus on this component, only the literature on the GSR will be mentioned, brought to date with publications since 1965.

Parametric characteristics of habituation of the OR

1. 'Given that a particular stimulus elicits a response, repeated applications of the stimulus result in decreased response (habituation). The decrease is usually a negative exponential function of the number of stimulus presentations.'

The response decrement was first clearly demonstrated by Davis (1934) and has repeatedly been confirmed in later studies. With ten presentations of a tone of 800 cps, 98 db, duration 2 sec, repeated every 48 sec, Davis, Buchman and Frankmann (1955) found a distinctly decreased response.

Dykman, Reese, Galbrecht and Thomasson (1959) likewise used tones, 800 cps, 60 db, duration 5 sec, presented at one minute intervals. They, too, obtained a clearly decreasing response, particularly on the first few trials. Similar results, under the same conditions, were obtained by Galbrecht, Dykman, Reese and Suzuki (1965).

Kimmel and Kimmel (1965) have demonstrated decreased response on repeated presentations of visual stimuli. A light stimulus (intensity unknown) with a duration of 1 sec was repeated every 20 or 30 sec; the total number of presentations was 10.

Another point concerns the nature of the habituation curve, which reportedly is a negative exponential function. The applicability of this quantitative model can be studied in two ways. First, by measuring whether the ratio of each successive pair of responses is constant. Secondly, by taking the logarithm of the function, which should generate a linear function. If the original function was

$y = a \cdot e^{-x}$, the new function becomes

$\log y = \log a - (\log e)x$, which shows that log y is a linear function of x (x represents the stimulus number and y the response amplitude).

Now the remarkable fact is that Montagu and Coles (1966) maintain that a linear relation exists between the response amplitude (change in log conductance) and the logarithm of the stimulus number. Mathematically, this statement is incompatible with the previous one, since substitution of log x for x in the function $y = a \cdot e^{-x}$ does not generate a linear function.

Unlike Thompson and Spencer, Montagu and Coles have clearly indicated their response measure, so that more rigorous testing is possible.

2. 'If the stimulus is withheld, the response tends to recover over time (spontaneous recovery).'

This is a very general characteristic; the literature will be discussed under the next point (3). The time required for spontaneous recovery apparently depends on several variables, so that it can hardly be regarded as characteristic of habituation.

3. 'If repeated series of habituation training and spontaneous recovery are given, habituation becomes successively more rapid.'

Thompson and Spencer propose the term 'potentiation of habituation' to describe this phenomenon. The suggestion is superfluous, however, since the term intersession habituation is already in use; by contrast, habituation within one stimulus series is called intrasession habituation. It will be clear that if intersession habituation can be demonstrated, this will implicitly apply also to spontaneous recovery.

Another point is that intersession habituation occurs not only after spontaneous recovery, but also after dishabituation brought about by another stimulus. The phenomenon as such was first demonstrated by Davis (1934). Rachman (1960) was able to demonstrate intersession habituation even after 6–8 weeks.

Galbrecht, Dykman, Reese and Suzuki (1965) found the effect after a 2 to 3 day interval. Intersession habituation after dishabituation was demonstrated by Zimny and Schwabe (1965), who used 8 presentations of a standard tone of 500 cps, 86 db, and then presented a single test tone of 1000 cps, 67 db or 4000 cps, 82 db. After this the original standard tone was presented 8 times again, followed by the 1000 cps or 4000 cps test tone, etc., until the test tone had been presented 4 times in all. A comparison of the responses to the first and the second test of 8 standard tones shows clearly that intersession habituation has occurred. This likewise applies to the responses to the various test tones.

4. 'Other things being equal, the more rapid the frequency of stimulation, the more rapid and/or more pronounced is habituation.'

Coombs (1938) found that an interval of 15 sec between tone stimuli produced more rapid habituation than a 30 sec interval. Geer (1966) used a tone stimulus of 1000 cps, 65 db, duration 2 sec. For three different groups the average interval was 20, 60 or 105 sec. The experiment showed that habituation decreased systematically with increasing intervals.

5. The rate of habituation depends on stimulus duration.

Although Thompson *et al.* do not mention stimulus duration as a variable, several studies have demonstrated the need for its inclusion. According to Sokolov (1963[b]), short stimuli habituate more quickly than long ones, but very long stimuli again produce rapid habituation. Sokolov, incidentally, gives no exact figures. Koepke and Pribram (1966) determined habituation rates for tones of 2 sec and 20 sec duration. While habituation to the 20 sec tones was a little slower, the difference was not significant.

6. 'The weaker the stimulus, the more rapid and/or more pronounced is habituation. Strong stimuli may yield no significant habituation.'

There is apparently one exception to this rule, namely, where threshold stimuli are concerned. According to Sokolov (1963[b]) threshold stimuli are very resistant to habituation. To date, as far as is known, this finding has not been confirmed in the West.

7. 'The effects of habituation training may proceed beyond the zero or asymptotic response level.'

Continuing stimulus presentations after complete habituation has been attained reportedly produce slower recovery. Thompson *et al.* consider this phenomenon a special case of the relation between the number of stimulus presentations and the degree of habituation.

8. 'Habituation of a response to a given stimulus exhibits stimulus generalization to other stimuli.'

Coombs (1938) demonstrated this phenomenon for auditory stimuli, while Porter (1938) found intersensory habituation, *viz.* from auditory to visual stimuli. On the other hand, habituation is never completely generalized. Its complement is dishabituation. The two phenomena are inversely proportional. Dishabituation will be dealt with separately.

9. 'Presentation of another (usually strong) stimulus results in recovery of the habituated response (dishabituation).'
10. 'Upon repeated application of the dishabituatory stimulus, the amount of dishabituation produced habituates (this might be called habituation of dishabituation).'

Discussion of the parametric characteristics mentioned under 9 and 10 must be deferred since these fall into the dishabituation category.

Thompson and Spencer always approach response decrement in terms of decreased amplitude of the response. Alternatively, however, such other response characteristics as latency and response duration can be considered. By response latency we understand the time elapsing between the onset of the stimulus and the onset of the response. By response duration is understood the time elapsing between the onset of the response and the moment at which it attains its maximum strength.

In the above mentioned experimental study of Koepke and Pribram (1966) it was found that during habituation a significant increase in response latency and a significant decrease of response duration took place.

Wolfensberger and O'Connor (1967), on the other hand, observed that the response latency was not significantly affected by stimulus repetition. (Nor, for that matter, was the response latency found to be dependent on stimulus duration, but it did show an inversely proportional relation to the stimulus intensity.)

Response duration, on the other hand, clearly proved to be a function of stimulus repetition, as well as to depend on stimulus duration and intensity. The amplitude measure was found to occupy an intermediate position: while it was dependent on stimulus repetition and intensity, it was not dependent on stimulus duration. The authors also computed intercorrelations of the various response measures, but no exact data are given. The highest correlations were found to exist between latency and amplitude, the lowest between latency and duration. In general, the correlations were somewhat higher with shorter stimulus duration.

3.3 THEORIES OF HABITUATION

A sound theory of habituation will not be confined to accounting for habituation phenomena but will also have to deal with dishabituation. Sokolov (1960), for instance, found that if after habituation of the OR to a tone the intensity of that tone was lowered while all other conditions remained unchanged, the OR reappeared. He concluded from this that habituation cannot be some fatigue-like process. Any perceptible change in stimulation will result in dishabituation. It is therefore natural to assume that the incoming signal is compared with a kind of standard.

Over the years a number of models have been proposed to account for habituation. Lynn (1966) distinguishes two kinds, 'one-stage models' and 'two-stage models'. The supporters of the one-stage model, among them Pavlov, Roitbak, Sharpless, Jasper and Gastaut, assume (to quote Lynn) that 'when a particular body of neurones is continually stimulated, an inhibitory process is generated in these neurones which raises their threshold of response'. This inhibition is supposed to be responsible for the habituation phenomena.

The one-stage models, however, have proved untenable, since they can hardly, if at all, account for the dishabituation phenomena. Characteristically, the two-stage models assume a separate phase in which the stimulus is analyzed. The result of this analysis determines whether in a second phase excitatory or inhibitory mechanisms are set in train to evoke or suppress the OR. The most fully elaborated model (until recently) was Sokolov's, but Moruzzi and Jouvet have also done work in this direction (Sokolov's model will be extensively discussed in the next section). Like Sokolov, the two last mentioned authors state as their opinion that stimulus analysis probably occurs at the cortical level, but they differ as to the nature of the inhibitory mechanism. Since the subject is not relevant to our purpose, we shall refrain from further discussion.

Lynn (1966) has given a survey of the various views held on this issue. Although the explanatory powers of Sokolov's model are considerable, particularly as regards dishabituation by weaker stimuli, it has certain flaws. Thus Thompson and Spencer (1966) point out that there is no strict logical necessity to postulate a process in which stimuli are compared with stimulus models.

Hind *et al.* (1961) found that certain neurons respond to weak tones and others to strong ones. Thompson and Spencer suggest that this finding makes Sokolov's stimulus model superfluous. The only assumption that needs to be made is that synaptic activity decreases as a result of stimulus repetition. Any other stimulus to a greater or less extent activates different neurons whose synaptic activity has not yet decreased. Thompson and Spencer therefore arrive at this conclusion: 'Dishabituation by change to a weaker or otherwise altered stimulus then becomes an instance of incomplete stimulus generalization of habituation. A stimulus having somewhat different central connections than the habituating stimulus yields a larger net response because generalization of habituation to the new stimulus is only partial.' The authors believe that they can adduce sufficient neurophysiological evidence for the decrease in synaptic activity. It is noteworthy that the results of Hind *et al.* (1961) concerning auditory stimulus analysis can be fully accommodated within this theory (Thompson was one of Hind's associates).

Sokolov's model, however, is not confined to auditory stimuli and, moreover, takes into account the temporal properties of the stimulation.

Stein (1966) criticizes Sokolov's theory on the grounds that such 'a hypothesis assumes as much as it explains'. The time required to scan the memory content (including stimulus models) would necessarily become progressively longer as the organism grows older, since the memory content increases as new models are being added. This conclusion seems erroneous to us since Sokolov (1963[b]) clearly stated that established stimulus models disappear again once the stimulus is no longer presented. Stein has proposed a different model, based on the principles of classical conditioning. He falls in with Sokolov's (1960) view that the excitatory system is activated by the onset of the novel stimulus and the inhibitory system by its prolongation, but assumes that the stimulus activates the excitatory system, which in its turn engages the inhibitory system. Stein further assumes that the activity of the inhibitory system is conditionable, in the Pavlovian sense, to the onset of the stimulus. The onset of the stimulus is thus regarded as the CS, the excitatory process as the UCS and the inhibitory process as the UCR. Stimulus repetition means reinforcement of the CS–UCR relation, so that excitation is increasingly counteracted by inhibition. The resultant of these last two processes manifests itself as phasic arousal, at least as long as excitation still dominates. In principle, therefore, both processes (excitation and inhibition) remain present, but as a result of conditioning the inhibitory process occurs more and more quickly and increasingly suppresses excitation. Upon complete habituation arousal disappears.

It is clear that if a novel stimulus is presented, excitation will again dominate at first, resulting in an arousal response (dishabituation). If some degree of stimulus similarity exists, there will be stimulus generalization of the inhibitory process, so that little or no arousal will result.

It is thus possible to explain dishabituation as a result of stimulus change. In this context spontaneous recovery is a matter of extinction of the established CR.

An important advantage of this theory is that it accounts for the 'below zero' habituation that can be observed in the form of a slower spontaneous recovery. After the arousal response has disappeared, the conditioning process with respect to the inhibitory system can continue, since the excitation (UCS!) is in fact still present. It follows that the extinction and consequently the spontaneous recovery of the arousal response will take longer. Stein likewise locates the excitatory system in the brainstem (RF); there is less certainty as to the anatomical substitute of the inhibitory system.

Stein's theory, however, is open to the same objection that it does not account for the effect of changes in the temporal properties of stimuli. Since Sokolov's theory, which is known as the 'neuronal model of the stimulus' is most fully developed and has provided the background for the present study, it will be discussed in a separate section.

3.4 THE NEURONAL MODEL OF THE STIMULUS

The model as such has been developed by Voronin and Sokolov (1960). Sokolov (1960) gives this definition:

> 'By neuronal model is meant a certain cell system whereby the information is stored concerning the properties of a stimulus which has been applied many times.'

These stimulus properties also include such temporal aspects as onset, duration and interval. Shortening of the stimulus duration will, according to Sokolov, elicit an OR at the moment when the stimulus formerly ended. The reverse will occur if the stimulus is prolonged. In that case an OR may be expected at the moment when the stimulus exceeds its original duration. In more general terms, an OR will be generated whenever the stimulus being presented no longer matches the neuronal model of the stimulus. This also applies to the temporal order of stimulation. As a result of omission of a stimulus from a sequence, or of changes within complex or compound stimuli, the incoming signal will fail to match the model.

Because of the selective nature of habituation, Sokolov regards the neuronal model as being in the nature of a selective filter. The properties of this filter can be studied by varying the stimulation parameters. The location of the filters must be at the cortical level since in decorticated animals the OR hardly habituates.

If the excitation-inhibition equilibrium at the cortical level shifts in the direction of inhibition (*e.g.* at the onset of sleep) the habituation effects are suppressed.

Shifts in the opposite direction reactivate habituation. Also, it is improbable that analysis of higher order stimuli (*e.g.* words) can take place at any but the cortical level. Physiologically, Sokolov (1960) proposes the following – diagrammatic – habituation model (fig. 3.1.).

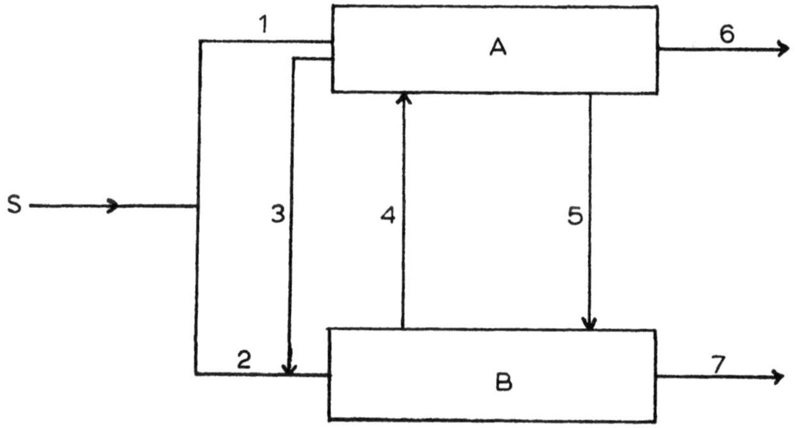

Fig. 3.1. Sokolov's habituation model

The sensory input (S) is transmitted in two ways, via the specific pathways (1) to the cortical level (A), and via the collaterals (2) to the reticular formation (B). A novel stimulus will activate B via pathway (2) and via pathways (1) and (5). The latter represents the cortico-reticular pathways through which excitatory impulses reach the RF. Activation of B elicits the autonomic and somatic components of the OR via (7). At the same time activation of the cortical level takes place via (4). The specific input is transmitted via (6). As a result of stimulus repetition, a stimulus model becomes established in A, producing negative feedback via (3) which blocks impulses traveling to B via (2). In other words, habituation is initiated. If, on the other hand, no neuronal model of an incoming stimulus exists or if the stimulus is appreciably different from a recently established model, an OR is elicited.

Sokolov (1960) regards the process whereby inhibition of the sensory input is brought about via (3) as the generation of a conditioned reflex. On this view, the onset of the stimulus acts as the CS for the prolongation of the stimulus which causes the inhibition (UCS). The conditional signal, Sokolov argues, sets in train the conditioned inhibition via the specific pathways (1) probably by hyperpolarization of the synaptic connections. He assumes that impulse transmission proceeds more rapidly in the specific system than along the non-specific pathways. The fact, however, that after habituation the OR reappears if the stimulus is withheld, cannot be explained from conditioned inhibition. This incongruity is ascertained by the neuronal model in A, which then sends down excitatory impulses to the RF via pathway (5).

In summary, the neuronal model of the stimulus has the following properties:

a) After repeated presentation of a constant stimulus the model comes to match the stimulus parameters within certain limits that are of the same order of magnitude as the just noticeable difference (j.n.d.).
b) After repeated stimulation with stimuli varying within certain limits the model is generalized in line with the limits of the stimulus variation.
c) The model is multidimensional (intensity, quality and temporal structures).
d) Complex stimuli (belonging to more than one modality) are likewise represented by a neuronal model.
e) Records are fixed in the neuronal model, not only of sensory but also of 'higher' properties of the stimulation (variables of meaning).

Habituation, however, is not permanent, but disappears over time. Further elaboration of the model will be required to account for this 'fading', or rather, considering its conditioned character, this extinction of habituation. To provide an explanation at the cellular level Sokolov (1963[a]) assumes that there are three types of neurons:

a) *afferent neurons:* these always respond to a stimulus, even with repeated presentation.
b) *extrapolatory neurons:* characteristically, these respond only if they have been activated before (reinforcement through repetition) and generate a sequence of impulses which anticipates the future impulse (before the next impulse is actually presented).
c) *comparator neurons:* these respond proportionally to the difference between the afferent and the extrapolatory neurons. In other words, if there is no difference, they do not respond.

The habituation process is assumed to proceed as follows. A record of the afferent signals is fixed in the extrapolatory neurons by a molecular mechanism. The extrapolatory neurons increasingly generate a sequence of impulses which anticipates future stimuli (an elementary form of conditioning at the cellular level). As soon as the impulse patterns of the afferent and the extrapolatory neurons come to match, the comparator neurons cease their activity and habituation is complete.

Neurophysiological evidence for the existence of these types of neurons has been obtained by means of micro-electrodes (extracellular). A survey of investigations in this field has been given by Sokolov (1966[a]) and Vinogradova (1966). Both types of neurons – extrapolatory and comparator – (sometimes called 'novelty detectors' or 'attention units') have been found in the hippocampus.

The various OR components exhibit temporal differences in habituation. The autonomic components habituate more quickly than the central components, *i.e.*, the components of the respective analyzers. This means that first the autonomic components are inhibited from the cortex, after which the cortex itself is inhibited. This latter inhibition, however, decreases cortex control of the RF, with the result that the OR will reappear after some time. If now the cortex is reactivated, for instance by some extraneous signal, the earlier habituation will return, once again blocking the OR to the original stimulus. The 'fading' of habituation, spontaneous recovery, is caused by chemical dissociation in the molecular mechanism of the extrapolatory neurons.

3.5 EXPERIMENTAL EVIDENCE FOR SOKOLOV'S MODEL

Allen, Hill and Wickens (1963) have shown that a change in a compound stimulus after habituation produces dishabituation. The stimulus consisted of three components, a visual stimulus (neon light) of 0.1 sec, a weak visual stimulus of 0.6 sec and a tone (1000 cps, 60 db) of 1.3, 1.05 or 0.75 sec. Three other groups received the tone before the weak visual stimulus. Each of the six experimental conditions thus presented a somewhat different compound stimulus. After ten stimulus presentations only the tone or the weak visual stimulus was presented. This change produced a significant increase of the GSR.

Sokolov (1960) investigated the filter properties of the model and arrived at the conclusion that the degree of dishabituation is a monotonically increasing function of the distance between the original stimulus and the new stimulus. In his experiment Sokolov habituated the OR to a 1000 cps tone by repeating the stimulus. His OR indicator was the number of seconds of alpha-rhythm blocking. After complete habituation – absence of any alpha blocking – the generalization of habituation to tones of 250, 500, 2000, 4000 and 8000 cps was studied in the form of dishabituation and measured in terms of duration of alpha blocking.

The following values were found. For 500 and 2000 cps (renewed) alpha blocking was 7.5 sec, for 250 and 4000 cps 11 and 10.3 sec respectively, while for 8000 cps (renewed) alpha blocking lasted 10.7 sec. The values for 500 and 2000 cps are thus the same; each of these tones differs one octave from the original tone. The tones of 250 and 4000 cps, each at two octaves' distance from the original tone, show alpha blocking of 11 and 10.3 sec respectively. The 8000 cps tone with 10.7 sec does not fit well into this picture.

Differences of one and two octaves from the original stimulus both produce an effect that is independent of the direction of the difference. In both directions the effect of two octaves' difference is nearly 1.5 sec more than that of the octave. Plotting the obtained values in a curve produces the 'filter model', or in other words, a representation of the filter properties of the neuronal model of the stimulus.

Kimmel (1960) conducted an experiment in which also a kind of filter curve was obtained. His objective was to determine whether the size of the perceptual disparity response (PDR) is a function of the size and/or direction of the discrepancy between expected and actual stimuli. It may be argued that this problem is essentially one of generalization of habituation. The stimulus which has been habituated is, from the subject's point of view, more likely to occur than any other stimulus. The PDR measured as an OR will then be a function of the degree of discrepancy (= stimulus disparity) between the two stimuli.

Kimmel's experiment, which among other things included GSR conditioning, proceeded as follows.

Subjects successively received: the CS (3 ×), the test stimulus TS (3 ×), the UCS (shock) (3 ×), the CS (6 ×), 20 acquisition trials (CS-UCS), and the TS (6 ×). Only the first TS of the last group was taken into account.

Table 3.1 Differences between test stimulus and conditional stimulus

CS\TS	45 db	75 db	105 db
35 db	+ 10	+ 40	+ 70
55 db	− 10	+ 20	+ 50
75 db	− 30	0	+ 30
95 db	− 50	− 20	+ 10
115 db	− 70	− 40	− 10

All CS's and TS's were 1000 cps; their duration was 4 sec. The CS intensities were 35, 55, 75, 95 and 115 db; the TS intensities were 45, 75 or 105 db. The table above (3.1) sets out these experimental conditions.

The figures in the cells indicate the difference in (db) intensity between the CS and the TS (Δ I).

Kimmel argued that the difference between the first TS after acquisition and the CS would determine the size of the PDR. This effect can be ascertained in two directions: for TS > CS and for TS < CS.

The table shows that the (Δ I) range runs from —70 db to +70 db in steps of 10 db. The (absolute) values in this range therefore indicate the degree of stimulus disparity.

Now the response to the TS cannot simply be used as the dependent variable (dependent on the stimulus disparity) if the intensity is manipulated as a stimulus dimension, since the absolute intensity of the stimulus itself to some extent determines the size of the response. Individual differences in responsivity likewise affect response size.

To control for these effects Kimmel determined for each subject the difference between the GSR to the TS and the mean of the GSR's to the three presentations of the TS prior to the acquisition phase. This difference was regarded as the PDR. If the PDR's thus computed are now plotted against the corresponding values of ΔI, a kind of filter curve is obtained which shows that the PDR is indeed a function of the value and direction of ΔI. PDR dependence on the direction of ΔI was demonstrated by the lower outcomes for negative ΔI's than for positive ΔI's.

Kimmel's method is open to serious objections. First of all, the question arises whether the response to the first TS (TS_1) in the extinction phase is not in part determined by generalization of the conditioned response to CS towards TS. Kimmel thinks that this is not the case, but his method for demonstrating absence of conditioning for intensities above 40 db has been shown to be inadequate (Orlebeke, van Olst, 1968).

Briefly, his method for eliminating individual differences is to express each response (in this case the CR) as a proportion of the first set of responses to the unpaired CS. If, however, groups are used which receive different CS intensities, this method does not work. Since the response to the CS is a function of the CS intensity, the corrected responses of the different groups are not comparable. Under conditions that are otherwise identical the relative responses will, by definition, become smaller if the CS intensity increases. This, however, is quite unrelated to the conditioning.

Another point, which has been made before, is that if the stimulus is of relatively short duration, the various GSR components cannot be distinguished.

A second, related, criticism is that omission of the UCS after conditioning also evokes a GSR. While it may be assumed that this effect is probably more or less constant for all experimental conditions (van Olst, Orlebeke, 1966[b]), the filter curve will nevertheless have shifted.

Finally, it may be asked to what extent habituation – the TS had already been presented three times prior to the acquisition trials – and sensitization by the UCS have played a part. In view of these drawbacks it is not advisable to use this method in investigating stimulus disparities.

Bernstein (1968) has studied the effect of the direction of stimulus change with changing stimulus intensity. One group received a tone of 60 db (1000 cps), another of 90 db (1000 cps). After habituation both groups received a test tone of 75 db (1000 cps). The amplitude of the dishabituation response in the +15 db group (60 → 75 db) was significantly larger than in the —15 db group (90 → 75 db). Apart from the stimulus change as such, the absolute intensity of the stimulation apparently plays a part in dishabituation as well.

Zimny and Schwabe (1965) have tested eight hypotheses derived from Sokolov's theory. In their experiment 36 standard stimuli (SS's) of 500 cps, 86 db were presented. Four interpolations of a test stimulus (TS) were made; a 1000 cps TS (67 db) for one group and a 4000 cps TS (82 db) for another group. The interstimulus interval was 20, 30 or 40 sec, at random. After eight SS's the first TS was presented (TS_1); the second TS (TS_2) after SS_{16}, TS_3 after SS_{24} and TS_4 after SS_{32}.

The following hypotheses were formulated and tested:

1. 'Habituation of the OR to the SS occurs during the first set of presentations of the SS.'

Owing to the neuronal model becoming established, a response decrement will occur during presentation of the first eight SS's. The difference was measured between the mean of SS_1 and SS_2, and of SS_7 and SS_8. The difference was significant ($p < .005$).

2. 'Presentation of a TS produces a return of the OR.'

For the combined groups the difference in response amplitude was tested between each TS and the preceding SS. In all cases the significance level was $p < .005$.

3. 'The greater the dissimilarity between a TS and the SS, the greater is the return of the OR.'

The experimental data (TS_{1-4} both for 1000 cps and for 4000 cps) were subjected to an analysis of variance for repeated measures. While the trials effect was significant ($p < .025$), the difference between $TS_{1000\ cps}$ and $TS_{4000\ cps}$ was not.

4. 'The OR to the first SS following a TS is greater than that to the SS immediately preceding the TS.'

The neuronal model established by the one presentation of a TS may interact with the model of the SS, or, put another way, an interpolated stimulus will cause some degree of dishabituation, as a result of which the OR to the subsequent SS will be larger. For the combined groups the differences between the post-TS SS's and the pre-TS SS's were tested and found significant. The p values for the differences between post and pre-SS values were: TS_1 $p<.05$; TS_2 $p<.005$; TS_3 $p<.01$; TS_4 $p<.005$.

5. 'The greater the dissimilarity between a TS and the SS, the greater the difference between the OR to the SS preceding a TS and that to the SS following a TS.'

This hypothesis is a logical sequel to hypotheses 3 and 4. An analysis of variance for repeated measures was carried out to establish whether $TS_{4000\ cps}$ causes more dishabituation than $TS_{1000\ cps}$. The TS effect proved significant ($p<.025$).

6. 'The OR to the TS is greater than that to the SS immediately following the TS.'

Presentation of one TS will cause only partial dissociation of the neuronal model of the SS, so that on presentation of the next SS there will still be some degree of habituation. For the combined groups the differences between each TS and the succeeding SS were tested. All four differences proved to be significant. For TS_1, $p<.005$; for TS_2, $p<.05$; for TS_3, $p<.005$; for TS_4, $p<.05$.

7. 'The greater the dissimilarity between a TS and the SS, the less the drop in OR from the TS to the succeeding SS.'

A more dissimilar TS will cause more dishabituation and hence a larger OR to the SS, so that the drop from TS to SS is smaller.* Experimental testing of

* This argument does not appear to be entirely cogent. A more dissimilar TS will itself evoke a larger OR, at least theoretically. Only if a maximum response is assumed would hypothesis 7 appear to be meaningful.

the hypothesis yielded a significant result ($p < .05$). This could mean that the size of the OR to the TS is not after all a function of stimulus dissimilarity, which is in line with the experimental findings obtained in testing hypothesis 3.
8. 'Habituation of the OR occurs over repeated presentations of the TS.' Each presentation of the TS will likewise establish a neuronal model of the TS, with resulting habituation. An analysis of variance showed the trials effect (habituation) to be significant ($p < .025$).

Koepke and Pribram (1966) conducted an experimental study of the temporal properties of the neuronal model of the stimulus. A tone of 1000 cps, 94 db, duration 2 or 20 sec, was presented either every 10 or 30 sec or every 30 or 60 sec until habituated. Now the duration of the stimulus was reversed, from 2 sec to 20 sec, and from 20 sec to 2 sec.

About half the subjects were found to respond to the stimulus change. Latencies were analyzed to establish whether the response was in fact to the change in stimulus duration rather than to the stimulus onset. The results are given in table 3.2.

Table 3.2 Mean latencies in sec

	Stimulus duration	2 sec (a)	20 sec (b)
Lt	first response	2.5	2.5
	last response	3.2	3.8
	reversal response	4.9	5.3

Both reversals had a significant effect on the Lt ($p < .01$). (Lt is measured from the *onset* of the stimulus). If there has been a response to the change in duration, the Lt must at least be greater than 2 sec, since the change cannot be noticed until 2 sec after the onset of the stimulus. Habituation increases the Lt, but dishabituation will suppress this effect. It is reasonable to assume that the 'true' Lt will have a value lying between the Lt's of the first and last responses. To this must be added the above 2 sec. If the mean Lt is taken as an estimate of the 'true' Lt, the total Lt will be for

a. $$2 + \frac{2.5 + 3.2}{2} = 4.9$$

b. $$2 + \frac{2.5 + 3.8}{2} = 5.2$$

These values are in agreement with the obtained values of 4.9 and 5.3.

From the theory of the neuronal model Geer (1967) has derived the hypothesis that the precision of the model is a function of the number of stimulations. This would be evidenced by an increase of the difference between the response to the standard stimulus and to the test stimulus with an increasing number of presentations of the standard stimulus. Geer reports an experiment in which after 5 or 15 presentations of the standard stimulus the test stimulus was presented (*i.e.* on the 6th or 16th trial). The difference between the 15th and 16th trials was significantly greater than that between the 5th and 6th trials ($p < .025$). On the other hand, the difference between trials 6 and 16 was not significant. This only means, however, that after 15 trials there is more habituation than after 5 trials.

In this experiment with tone stimuli the standard stimulus was of 2 sec duration, while the test stimulus was 12 sec. At the same time Geer tested a second hypothesis, concerning latency, stating that if the subject responds to the change in stimulus duration, the latency of the response to the novel stimulus must exceed the Lt to the preceding stimulus, the increase in the Lt being more pronounced if the stimulus model is more established. The experimental findings confirmed both the Lt lengthening ($p < .01$) and the difference in Lt between the 6th and 16th trials ($p < .05$). The average increase in Lt from the 15th to the 16th trial was 1.9 sec. The conclusion can be drawn that subjects did actually respond to the change in stimulus duration. It may be noted that these last findings concur with the above results of Koepke and Pribram.

The neuronal model also provides fixation of other than sensory parameters of the stimulus. Unger (1964) has demonstrated that stimuli from a non-sensory dimension can likewise be studied by means of a psychophysiological indicator (dishabituation of the OR). Unger's approach is in line with the views of *e.g.* Sharpless and Jasper (1956), who use the term 'stimulus specificity' in habituation to denote the fact that even a slight change in stimulation will cause dishabituation. While Sharpless and Jasper confine this stimulus specificity to the repetition of physically identical stimuli, Unger endeavors to place habituation within a wider framework. The stimuli used by him are the natural numbers 1, 2, 3, etc. Naturally, these stimuli are not physically identical. To the subject, however, such a series represents a logically ordered whole, causing him to anticipate strongly the subsequent terms of the series, or, in other words, a certain pattern of expectation is established. Undoubtedly more complex processes are involved than in the presentation of single tones.

Unger has attempted to answer the question whether 'higher order' stimuli of this kind are also amenable to the habituation and dishabituation process. His subjects received the numbers 1, 2, 3 etc. in their normal order, at intervals of from 5 to 25 seconds, depending on the state of the response system. The response measured was the vasomotor component of the OR, *i.e.* vasoconstriction in the finger. The habituation criterion was absence of response to the numbers 14, 15 and 16. Instead of the expected 17 another 15 was presented. If habituation was delayed, subjects received a 29 instead of 27. The results showed that in spite of marked interindividual and intraindividual variability 12 out of 20 subjects attained a habituation criterion followed by a pronounced OR on presentation of the 'novel' stimulus.

This experiment provides some evidence that stimuli belonging to a non-sensory dimension also conform to the rules of the model for habituation and dishabituation. A consequence is of course that the neuronal model of the stimulus must be linked with a memory capacity for storing information on the particular stimulus dimension. The present author has confirmed Unger's findings, using the GSR as dependent variable (unpublished paper).

3.6 HABITUATION AS A FUNCTION OF SPONTANEOUS ACTIVITY

In principle, only stimulus properties have so far been discussed as determinants of habituation. It has been found, however, that habituation is influenced by still another factor, the so-called spontaneous activity. This spontaneous activity manifests itself as the occurrence of non-specific responses, *i.e.* responses not caused by demonstrable stimuli. The usual index for this activity is the number of spontaneous responses occurring during a certain length of time (a few minutes) immediately preceding one or more stimuli. The reliability of this index appears to be quite fair. Thus Johnson (1963) found in a replication after 48 hours a reliability of rho = .69 ($p < .01$) for spontaneous GSR activity.

Having established the median of spontaneous activity, Johnson divided his subjects into a stable (< md) and an unstable (> md) group. The unstable group clearly showed less habituation to tone stimuli (500 cps, 73 db, duration 5 sec, interval 55 sec) and alternating light stimuli. The above experiment of Koepke and Pribram (1966) likewise demonstrated a difference in habituation rate. The average rate of the stable group was 5.5 as against 19.0 for the unstable group; this difference was significant ($p < .02$). (The habituation rate is defined as the number of trials required to attain complete habituation).

Leavy and Geer (1967) found a correlation of $r = .51$ between spontaneous GSR activity and habituation rate ($p < .001$).

Geer (1967), studying the effect of interstimulus intervals on the correlation between spontaneous activity and habituation rate, computed the following correlations between these phenomena:

Interval	correlation	p
20 sec	$r = .001$	n.s.
60 sec	$r = .31$	n.s.
105 sec	$r = .44$	$p < .05$

The interval groups showed no significant differences as far as spontaneous activity was concerned. In the total group the correlation was $r = .22$ ($p < .05$).

PART II

AN INVESTIGATION OF SOME PROPERTIES AND FUNCTIONS OF THE OR

INTRODUCTION

In the first part a survey has been given of research on the OR and in particular on the GSR component of the OR. The field has by no means been explored in its entirety, while moreover the work done so far is incomplete in that

a) there have been few replications of experimental studies;
b) the stimulus variables have as a rule been varied over a narrow range;
c) it is difficult to interpret the work of Russian investigators because of the absence of statistical analyses and tests.

It is primarily against this background that the present investigation has been undertaken. Its central purpose is to obtain reliable quantitative information on the nature and function of the OR. Further research on the OR is conditional on the availability of this type of data. This is especially true of such applied subjects in the (clinical and nonclinical) psychology of individual differences as the ranking of individuals along psychophysiological dimensions, in which the obtained psychophysiological values are correlated with the psychological variables used in the diagnostic procedures. As we noted with respect to the investigation described in 1.2.8, psychophysiological variables such as habituation rate, spontaneous activity, response latency, response amplitude etc. are used in this type of research.

To date, however, little is known about the relations among these variables. Further information on this point is essential to permit the workers in the psychology of individual differences to carry out psychophysiologically oriented research in depth, particularly on the problem of whether certain patterns of psychophysiological variables are related to certain characteristics of the personality. Quantitative information about the parameters of the OR is also essential for studying the role of the OR in certain behavioral processes such as stimulus generalization, classical conditioning, skill learning, etc. Again, there is a need for further information about the quantitative relations (interdependence) between such different response measures as amplitude, duration and latency as well as about the trend of the pre-stimulus level. The experiments reported in this second part primarily deal with habituation and dishabituation of the OR in response to sensory and complex stimuli. The main questions that we have endeavored to answer are: what parameters determine the habituation process, and under what conditions does dishabituation occur? Within this general context we have tested some more specific hypotheses concerning such topics as the supposed linear relationship between the response amplitude and the log of the stimulus number in habituation, the representation of temporal stimulus properties in the neuronal model of the stimulus, and Sokolov's filter model for dishabituation. The experiments involved not only purely sensory stimuli but also complex stimuli.

In a separate chapter (7) we shall further deal with the relation between perceptual expectation and OR occurrence, the inhibitory function of the OR, and the determinants of signalization, especially in differential signalization. The problems and experimental conditions will be set out in detail in the appropriate places. In the next chapter (4) the experimental variables and setup will be discussed.

4 THE EXPERIMENTAL VARIABLES, SETUP AND MEASUREMENT TECHNIQUE

4.1 THE NATURE OF THE EXPERIMENTAL VARIABLES

4.1.1 The stimuli

a) *The sensory stimuli*
All the sensory stimuli were of the auditory type, *viz.* pure tones. Four stimulus properties – intensity, duration, tone frequency and interstimulus interval – were used as variables and their effect on such phenomena as habituation studied. Each variable was employed at different levels. Systematic variation of one of these variables after habituation permitted us to study the effect on dishabituation. The question we sought to answer was whether the size of these dishabituation effects varied so systematically as to be considered indicative of the stimulus relations involved. Within this design various specific hypotheses and problems, some of which have been mentioned before, were studied and tested.

b) *The non-sensory or complex stimuli*
By way of non-sensory, 'higher-order' stimuli, sequences of numbers or words were used. Each item in a sequence may be regarded as a stimulus, and all the stimuli as being associated in a particular manner, according to the rule of the sequence. This implies that the dimension along which these stimuli are ordered is of a logical or analytic nature. It would therefore be appropriate to describe these as logical or logically qualified stimuli. If words are used as stimuli, the underlying dimension along which the verbal stimuli are ordered is a particular meaning or relationship among meanings. Words might therefore be called symbolic or semantic stimuli.

4.1.2 The instruction

As a rule, the experiment was started with habituation followed by dishabituation of non-signal stimuli. Subjects were given the following general instruction. (Most subjects had some time previously been informed about the conditions of the forthcoming experiment.)

'As you have been told before, we are going to conduct an attention test. You will hear a number of tones through the earphones. You are not required to do anything except listen. Upon completion of the session you will be asked a few questions. Since it is very important that you should sit absolutely still, settle yourself in a comfortable position, but do not go to sleep. If unforeseen circumstances should arise, you can speak to me through the microphone. Have you any questions?'

Upon completion of the habituation-dishabituation phase the experiment was briefly interrupted to give further instructions concerning the more specific part of the experiment. Details of these instructions will be given in the appropriate place.

4.1.3 The response system

In principle it makes very little difference which OR component is chosen as the response. In practice the GSR is most commonly used because of its relatively high sensitivity. For reasons of convenience we have conformed to this practice.

The GSR may be regarded as a temporary change in the apparent electrical resistance of the skin. This resistance can be measured by applying a voltage V across two electrodes attached to the skin so that a current I is passed through the electrodes. In accordance with Ohm's law, $V = I \times R$, the resistance R equals the ratio of V to I. The effect of a stimulus may be to cause a temporary drop of R, variously known as the 'electrodermal reponse' (EDR), 'galvanic skin response' (GSR), etc. These terms, however, suggest more than can strictly be proved. A more neutral term like 'skin resistance response' (SSR) therefore seems preferable.

The value of R prior to a stimulus presentation is called the pre-stimulus level, while the post-stimulus level of R is the value attained at the moment of maximum response (see fig. 4.1).

R_1 = pre-stimulus level

R_2 = post-stimulus level

R_1–R_2 = response

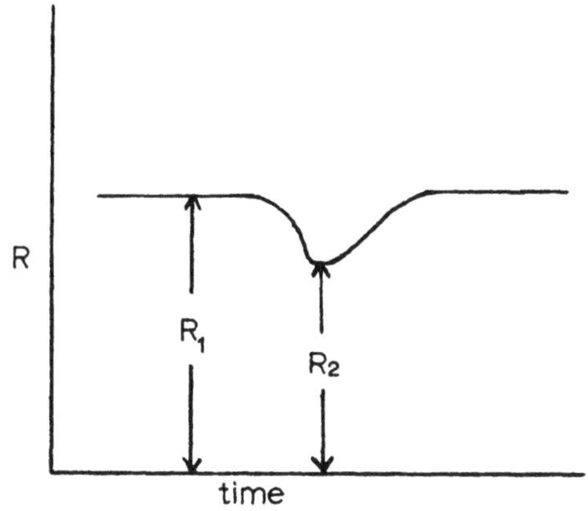

Fig. 4.1. Response wave of the GSR

Apart from amplitude, other response characteristics are latency (Lt), *i.e.* the time elapsing between the onset of the stimulus and the onset of the response, and response duration (Rd), the time elapsing between the onset of the response and the moment at which it attains its maximum amplitude. Little is known about the relation between these response variables. In various cases, Lt and Rd will therefore be used as response measures, in addition to amplitude.

Responses due to external stimuli are specific responses and show an Lt between 1.5 and 3.0 sec. Other, 'non-specific', responses may be regarded as due to non-identified stimuli or as a form of spontaneous activity in the response system.

No complete certainty exists about the physiological mechanism of the SRR. Edelberg (1967) concludes that by way of working hypothesis the SRR is to be regarded as 'an increase in the total permeability of a selective cutaneous membrane in response to the arrival of impulses carried by cholinergic sympathetic nerves'.

In general, two methods may be used for measuring the SRR; the method of constant current and the method of constant voltage. In the former case the variable measured is the voltage, which is a function of R, in the latter the current flow, which is a function of I/R or C (= conductance). In most cases the constant current method is used. The subject's resistance about to be measured is connected in series with a relatively large resistance, *e.g.* 1 M.Ohm

(= 10^6 Ohm). This circuit is linked up with a direct-current power supply, the voltage of which is so chosen as to keep the current density below 10 $\mu A/cm^2$. The current flow in this circuit is approximately constant. The voltage to be measured across the subject's resistance is, again approximately, proportional to this resistance.

The electrodes are an important part of the electrical circuit. A general condition is that the electrodes across which the voltage is measured must be nonpolarizing, *i.e.* the chemical composition of the electrodes must not be changed by the current flow. To this end a combination should be used of electrodes and an electrolyte which deposits the chemical equivalent of the electrodes. Frequently used are zinc electrodes in combination with zinc-sulphate (2.4% solution).

It is a well-known fact that the palm of the hand is a very 'active' area for the SSR. Maximization of the effect of this component can be achieved by attaching a small electrode to the palm of the hand and a large electrode to a 'passive' area, *e.g.* the forearm.*

The resistance is inversely proportional to the effective surface of the electrodes, so that a small electrode will make a relatively large contribution to the total resistance. It is advisable therefore to attach the small electrode to the 'active' area. Preferably, the 'active' electrode should be used as cathode, so that no zinc ions are driven into the skin. Zinc ions in the skin will affect the amplitude of the SSR. For further details we refer to van Olst and van der Ham (1967).

Another problem concerns the units in which the SRR is to be expressed. In view of what has been said above, the obvious choice would seem to be Ohms. In fact, this unit is not very suitable. The value of $R_1 - R_2$ depends very much on how large R_1 is, and R_1 varies a great deal between individuals. The problem is therefore to find a unit which shows little or no correlation with the pre-stimulus level.

Now, the change in resistance may equally well be considered a change in conductance (C), C being equal to 1/R. (C is expressed in Mho's or Siemens').

The response measured thus becomes the 'skin conductance response' (SCR). It has been demonstrated that $C_2 - C_1$ (= Δ C) is much less dependent on C_1.

* The resistance under the electrodes, *i.e.* between the surface and the underside of the skin constitutes practically the entire skin resistance; the resistance of the subcutaneous tissue, a few hundred Ohms, is negligible.

To facilitate manipulation, the unit adopted in practice is the µMho, rather than the Mho, which means that, if R is given, the value 1/R is multiplied by 10^6.

We may add that physiologically it is more meaningful to speak in terms of conductance and increased conductance since increased activity (arousal and arousal response) is accompanied by an increase in skin conductance. This is borne out by the finding of Thomas and Korr (1957) that conductance is a linear function of the number of active sweat glands according to the formula $C = N.m + C_0$, in which N is the number of active sweat glands and C_0 the conductance in the absence of sweat gland activity. C_0 has proved to be small and is frequently negligible; m is the conductance of one sweat gland.

Darrow (1937) has pointed out that psychological phenomena seldom show a linear correlation with biological functions. Biological systems tend to exhibit regularities of a logarithmic character. Darrow therefore proposed adopting the logarithm of conductance (log C) as response measure. This $\triangle$ log C, which is not to be confused with log $\triangle$ C, is held to show little correlation with the pre-stimulus level C_1.

Conversion of scores expressed in R can take place according to the rule:

$$\triangle \log C = \log R_1 - \log R_2,$$

which follows quite simply from

$$\begin{aligned}\triangle \log C &= \log C_2 - \log C_1\\ &= \log 1/R_2 - \log 1/R_1\\ &= \log R_1/R_2\\ &= \log R_1 - \log R_2\end{aligned}$$

In principle, $\triangle$ log C indicates the ratio C_2/C_1.

4.2 THE EXPERIMENTAL SETUP

Since the experiments were conducted outside the laboratory, an insulated, double-walled Amplifon unit (inside measurements 2 × 2 × 2 m) was used, which could be taken apart and reassembled. The unit was air-conditioned, so that a constant temperature of *c.* 20° C could be maintained. The subject was seated in an easy chair and the experimenter could communicate with him through a stereo amplifier.

The stimuli, all auditory, were presented through earphones. The pure tones were produced by a Philips audiometer, type A 06. The other stimuli were presented by means of a taperecorder. An electronic timer controlled duration and intervals in stimulus presentation.

Fig. 4.2

A: Subject
B: timer
C: recorder
D: 24-volt d-c power supply

R_1	=	200k ohm
R_2	=	10k ohm
R_3	=	1M ohm
R_4	=	10k ohm
R_5	=	1M ohm
R_6	=	50k ohm
R_7	=	10M ohm
R_8	=	10k ohm
R_9	=	1M ohm
R_{10}	=	100k ohm
R_{11}	=	*c.* 833 ohm
C_1	=	10 nF

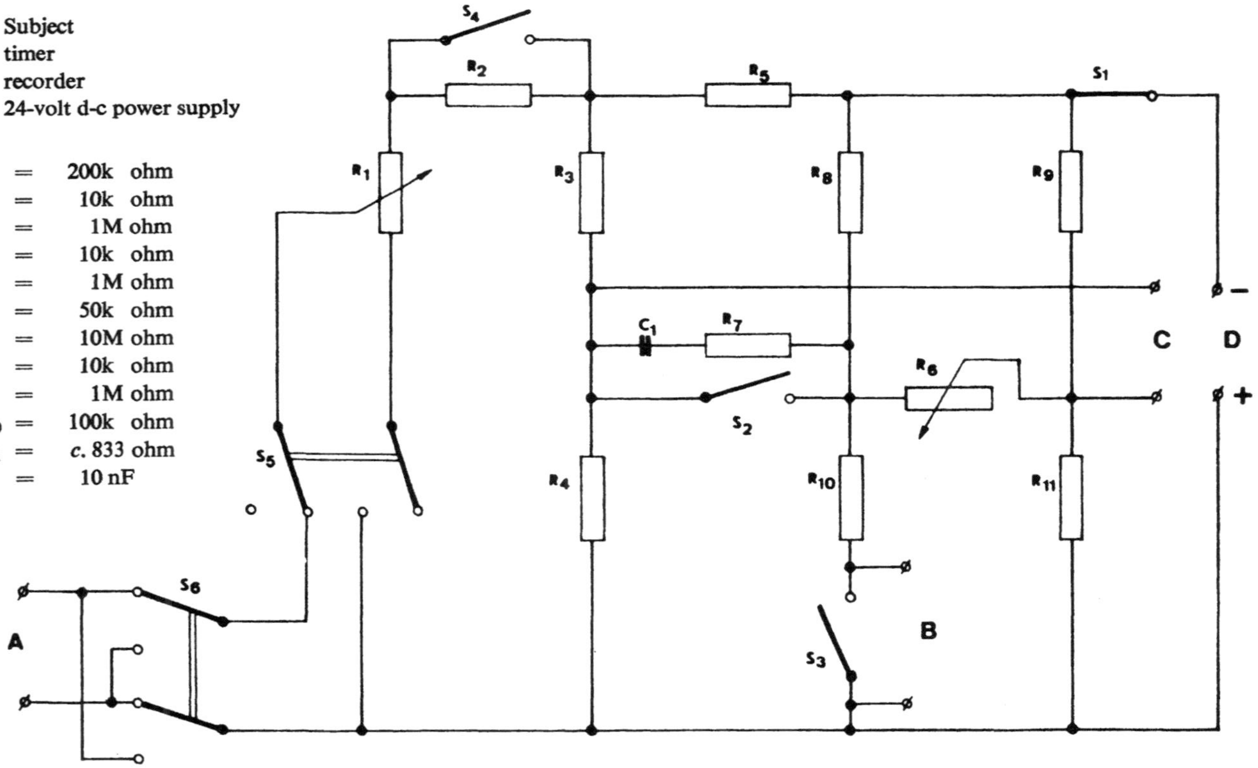

The response variable was the skin resistance measured by the method of constant current. The current intensity was 20 to 24 μA, which resulted in a density of 7 to 8 μA/cm². The electrical circuit is shown diagrammatically in fig. 4.2.

When S_5 is switched, the bridge can be brought into equilibrium by maximizing R_1 which at the same time sets the zero point of the scale. R_{11} is adjusted in such a way that the voltages across C is exactly zero (adjustment control). To this end, the combination of S_2 and R_6 is used as sensitivity control.

If S_4 is now closed, the resistance in the arm in which the subject's resistance will be recorded decreases by 1 K Ohm (R_2). This change produces a certain deflection, which will be used for calibrating later deflections. S_5 is now reset, so that the subject is connected to the measurement device. By means of R_1 the bridge is again brought into equilibrium.

R_1 is in the form of a decade switch with steps of 20 K Ohms. The position of R_1 determines the upper and lower limits of the scale on the recorder. The combination of R_7, R_8, R_{10} and C_1 serves to mark the start of the stimulus on the recorder. (The recorder used had only one channel, which also had to serve for stimulus marking.) If S_3 is closed for a moment, a small peak will appear in the base line registered by the recorder. In regular stimulus sequences this circuit via B was controlled by the timer.

Since the voltage across D is 24 V, the current flow I equals

$$\frac{24}{R_1 + R_5} = \frac{24}{1{,}2 \times 10^6} = 20\ \mu A.$$

This value, which produced a current density of 7 to 8 μA/cm² on the 'active' electrode (surface *c.* 3 cm²), was chosen, first, to ensure minimal polarization effects and, secondly, to prevent the skin potentials (Tarchanoff phenomenon) from producing a disturbing effect (Venables and Martin, 1967). By means of the commutator S_6, which reverses the direction of the current, one can check whether polarization has taken place.

The electrodes had the following characteristics. The small electrode (cathode), attached to the palm, consisted of a small plastic cylinder, 1.5 cm high, 3 cm² across, closed at the top. A zinc strip was attached to the inside of the top cover, and the rest of the space was taken up by a cylinder-shaped piece of sponge soaked in $ZnSO_4$ 2.4‰. The passive electrode (anode), attached to the outside of the wrist, consisted of an oblong zinc strip, 45 cm² large, on top of a piece of sponge of the same dimensions, likewise soaked in

$ZnSO_4$ 2.4%. Both electrodes were held in place by nylon adhesive tape.

Registration took place by means of a Speedomax H Compact Azar, manufactured by Leeds and Northrup. (A millivolt-recorder adjustable as regards both range and zero point.)

RT measurement

In a number of cases reaction times were measured by means of an electric stopwatch (Jacquet) which gave readings in 0.01 sec. Reaction times always concerned responses to single stimuli produced by the above audiometer (and presented through headphones). For further details see Ch 5.3.1and 5.4.

Subjects

In all, 350 subjects were used, varying in age from 16 to 20. Their average educational level was three or four years of secondary modern school or trade school.

5 AN INVESTIGATION OF THE OR AND OR HABITUATION AS A FUNCTION OF VARIOUS SENSORY STIMULUS PARAMETERS

In this chapter the following relations will be studied by analysis of the collected data:

a) The OR as a function of the levels of the various stimulus parameters (2, 3, 4)
b) The relations between the various response measures (8)
c) The relation between the response amplitude and the pre-stimulus level (10)
d) OR habituation as a function of the levels of the various stimulus parameters, of the magnitude of the first response and of the pre-stimulus level (1, 6, 7, 9, 11)
e) The shape of the habituation curve (5).

The numbers in brackets refer to the subdivisions in the general scheme of analysis (5.2.2) as well as to the actual analyses presented under the various stimulus parameters.

As stated before, the experimental study comprised four auditory stimulus parameters: duration, interval, tone frequency (pitch) and intensity, each at several levels. In each experimental condition presentation of the tone stimulus continued until no response occurred on three successive trials, with a maximum of twenty stimulations. Habituation rate is the number of stimulus presentations required for complete habituation. If on the nth trial no response occurs for the third successive time, the habituation rate is thus n-3.*

* The commonly used definition of habituation rate is liable to cause misunderstandings. If habituation proceeds more quickly, this manifests itself in a decrease of the number of trials, *i.e.* in a lower habituation rate. If, on the other hand, we say there is an increase in habituation rate, this means that the habituation process proceeds more slowly.

In the next section a survey will be given of the various stimulus conditions.

5.1 A SURVEY OF THE STIMULUS PARAMETERS (SEE ALSO TABLE 5.1)

I. *Stimulus duration*

Forty subjects (four groups of ten) received a tone of2000 cps and 59 db (standard reference is 2.10^{-4} microbar), repeated every 20 sec. For the first group the stimulus duration was 0.1 sec, for the second group 0.5 sec, for the third group 2.5 sec, and for the fourth group 12.5 sec.

II. *Stimulus-interval*

Forty subjects (four groups of 10) received a tone of 2000 cps, 59 db, duration 0.5 sec. For the first group the interstimulus interval was 5 sec, for the second group 10 sec, for the third group 20 sec, and for the fourth group 40 sec.

III. *Interaction between the duration and interval parameters*

A complementary experiment was conducted to study the possible interaction between the two previous parameters. Twenty subjects (two groups of 10) received a tone of 2000 cps, 59 db and a 5 sec interval. For the first group the duration was 0.1 sec, for the second group 2.5 sec.

IV. *Tone frequency*

Fifty subjects (five groups of 10) received tones of equal subjective loudness with a duration of 0.5 sec and an interval of 10 sec.

The first group a tone of 500 cps, 56 db.
The second group a tone of 1000 cps, 60 db.
The third group a tone of 2000 cps, 59 db.
The fourth group a tone of 4000 cps, 54 db.
The fifth group a tone of 8000 cps, 65 db.

These intensities were selected from the table of Robinson and Dadson (1957) for equal subjective loudness.

V. *Intensity*

Forty subjects (four groups of 10) received a tone of 2000 cps, duration 0.5 sec, at 10 sec intervals. For the first group the intensity was 39 db,

Table 5.1 A survey of the stimulus parameters

Stimulus parameter	Levels					Other characteristics
I Duration	0.1 sec	0.5 sec	2.5 sec	12.5 sec		2000 cps, 59 db, interval 20 sec
II Interval	5 sec	10 sec	20 sec	40 sec		2000 cps, 59 db, duration 0.5 sec
III Duration	0.1 sec	2.5 sec				2000 cps, 59 db, interval 5 sec
IV Tone frequency	500 cps	1000 cps	2000 cps	4000 cps	8000 cps	duration 0.5 sec, interval 10 sec
V Intensity	39 db	59 db	79 db	99 db		2000 cps, duration 0.5 sec, interval 10 sec

for the second group 59 db, for the third group 79 db and for the fourth group 99 db.

The table 5.1 sets out the stimulus variables. Each cell represents the experimental conditions of 10 subjects.

The results thus obtained were analyzed in a number of ways to answer the questions formulated in 5.2.2.

5.2 DATA PROCESSING AND ANALYSIS

5.2.1 Presentation of the data

The data for each stimulus parameter will be presented in a number of tables and figures.

Table A1: Mean response amplitude per stimulus presentation for the various levels of the particular stimulus parameter.

Table A2: Mean habituation rate for each level of the particular stimulus parameter.

Table A3: Mean latency of the first and last responses for each level of the particular stimulus parameter.

Table A4: Mean response duration of the first and last responses for each level of the particular stimulus parameter.

Table A5: Mean pre-stimulus level per stimulus presentation for the various levels of the particular stimulus parameter.

Fig. A1: The correlation between the mean response amplitude and the logarithm of the stimulus number.

In the presentation of the data per stimulus parameter the corresponding letter of the stimulus parameter will be added to the numbers.

5.2.2 General questions and methods of analysis

1 a) What is the effect of the various levels of a particular stimulus parameter on the habituation rate (HR)?

b) Since the maximum number of stimulations is twenty, there is a possibility that the measures do not completely fulfil the requirement of normal distribution. On the other hand, the number of observations is too small to permit a test for normality. By way of compromise we adopted the rule that if in a subgroup more than one HR = 20 occurred, the non-parametric analysis of variance of Kruskal and Wallis was applied. In all other cases a parametric analysis of variance was carried out.

2 a) What is the effect of the various levels of a particular stimulus parameter on the amplitude of the first response?
b) This question could be answered by a simple analysis of variance.

3 a) What is the effect of the various levels of a particular stimulus parameter on the latency of the first response?
b) See 2 b.

4 a) What is the effect of the various levels of a particular stimulus parameter on the response duration of the first response?
b) See 2 b.

5 a) Is there a linear relationship between the response amplitude and the logarithm of the stimulus number?
b) First the stimulus number y is transformed to the value z according to the rule $z = {}^2\log y + 1$. After transformation the original stimulus numbers 1, 2, 4 and 8 will thus be 1, 2, 3 and 4. The variance within this sequence, due to stimulus repetition, is now analyzed to find a linear component.

If the response amplitude is not affected by the level of the stimulus parameter (see question 2), the measures for each stimulus number are summated over the levels of stimulation. In this case an analysis of variance for repeated measures is carried out for three sources of variance: 'stimulus numbers', 'subjects' and the interaction between these two factors, which is made the 'error' term.

If the particular stimulus variable does affect the response amplitude, the stimulus level is introduced as a separate factor. In that case the analysis first determines the variances due to 'stimulus levels' and to 'subjects within the stimulus levels', which is made the 'error' term for the first source of variance. After that the variances due to 'stimulus numbers' and to the interaction between 'stimulus levels'and 'stimulus numbers' are determined. In both cases the 'error' term is the interaction between 'stimulus numbers' and 'subjects within the stimulus levels' (see Edwards, 1960, Ch 14).

In each case, therefore, the variance due to 'stimulus numbers' is analyzed to find a linear component. However, individuals as a rule differ so much in habituation rate that not all measures can be taken into account. Only those cases will be considered where the HR is 8 or more. If these cases exhibit a significant linear component, the function $y = -ax + b$ will also be determined, y being the response amplitude, x the stimulus number z, a the coefficient of direction and b the amplitude of the first response.

6 a) What is the effect of the habituation process on response latency (Lt)?

b) This problem can be treated by the same type of analysis of variance for repeated measures as has been discussed under 5b. The analysis first determines the variance due to levels of stimulation (A), the error term again being the variance of subjects within the stimulus levels (B). After that it determines the variances due to the habituation process (the difference between the first and the last response) (R) and the interaction $A \times R$. The 'error' term for both R and $A \times R$ is the interaction $B \times R$.

7 a) What is the effect of the habituation process on response duration (Rd)?

b) This problem is dealt with in the manner discussed under 6 b.

8 a) Does a relation exist between the response amplitude (Ra) and latency as well as between response amplitude and response duration (Rd)?

b) If, as a result of the habituation process, Lt and Rd undergo a change, there is in principle a possibility that this change is due to Lt and Rd dependence on Ra. While this is a likely assumption for response duration, latency may present a less clear picture. In both cases the correlation coefficient r between Lt and Ra as well as between Rd and Ra of the response to the *first* stimulus presentation will be computed.

9 a) What is the relation between the amplitude of the first response and the HR?

b) First it must be determined whether computation of Pearson's r is permitted. To this end a goodness-of-fit test for normality is carried out on the values of HR (Hays, 1963, Ch 17.3).
If there is too much deviation, the coefficient of rank correlation, rho, will be computed.

10 a) To what extent do the values of $\Delta \log C$ correlate with the pre-stimulus level?

b) To ensure a sufficient number of measures for this analysis, it will be carried out only if question 2 has been answered in the negative. The correlations will be computed for two cases, *viz.* for the first and the second response. The pre-stimulus level can be computed quite simply; $\log C_1 = 3 - \log R_1$ if R_1 is given in K Ohms. (Alternatively, calculation of the rank correlation between $\triangle \log C$ and C would suffice, although the chance that the null hypothesis, 'the correlation within this population is zero', can be rejected will be smaller in that case.)

11 a) Does a relation exist between the HR and the onset value of log C?

b) If analysis 9 has shown that the distribution of HR does not differ too much from the normal distribution, the correlation coefficient r will be computed for HR and log C (not to be confused with $\triangle \log C$). In general, the distribution of log C meets the requirement of normality of distribution better than does the distribution of C. If the distribution of HR shows too much deviation, the coefficient of rank correlation will be computed.

12 Finally, two questions remain, for which it is difficult to provide a general solution because of their descriptive character.

a) What changes occur in the pre-stimulus level as a result of stimulus repetition?

b) Are these changes related to the levels of stimulation?

The analyses are related to the tables in the following manner:

Analysis 1 relates to table A 2
Analysis 2 relates to table A 1 (trial 1)
Analysis 3 relates to table A 3 (a-values)
Analysis 4 relates to table A 4 (a-values)
Analysis 5 relates to figure A 1
Analysis 6 relates to table A 3
Analysis 7 relates to table A 4
Analysis 8 relates to table A 1, A 3 and A 4
Analysis 9 relates to table A 1 and A 2
Analysis 10 relates to table A 1 and A 5
Analysis 11 relates to table A 2 and A 5
Analysis 12 relates to table A 5

5.3 RESULTS

5.3.1 Stimulus duration

The various levels of stimulus duration are designated D_1, D_2, D_3 and D_4, representing 0.1, 0.5, 2.5 and 12.5 sec respectively.

Table A1D Mean response amplitude ($\triangle$ *log* C $\times$ 1000)

Data

Trials	Stimulus levels			
	D_1	D_2	D_3	D_4
1	24.7	23.6	21.4	35.4
2	19.9	8.9	6.2	9.6
3	15.7	5.3	5.6	10.5
4	12.0	2.8	2.6	5.7
5	9.6	2.5	4.2	4.8
6	5.8	3.7	3.9	4.6
7	3.6	1.3	1.1	6.1
8	4.3	0.9	1.8	2.9
9	0.9	0.6	1.1	2.5
10	1.0	1.1	1.3	4.3
11	5.7	0.7	3.1	2.5
12	2.4	2.1	0.3	1.5
13	1.9	0.0	0.5	3.1
14	1.3	0.1	0.4	2.5
15	1.2	0.6	0.0	2.1
16	0.7	0.7	0.6	3.6
17	1.0	0.2	0.4	3.5
18	1.1	0.8	0.4	1.5
19	1.1	0.8	0.2	1.2
20	1.0	0.3	0.1	4.0

Table A2D Mean habituation rate per stimulus level

Stimulus levels	D_1	D_2	D_3	D_4
Habituation rate	11.6	8.2	8.4	16.2

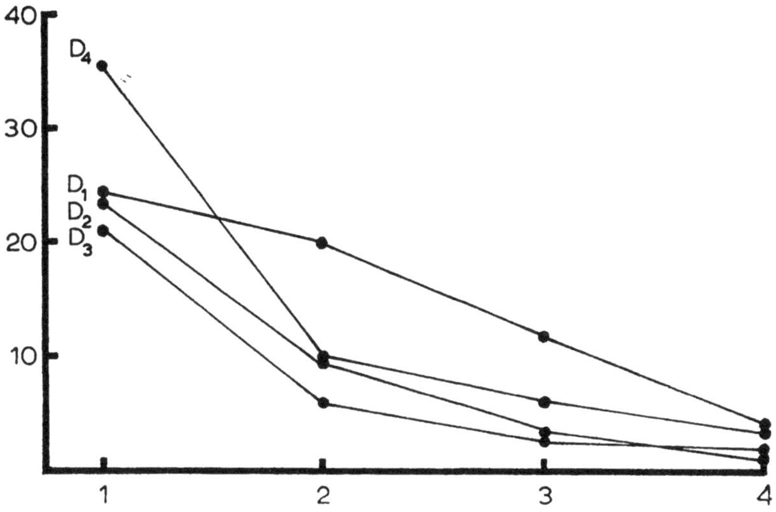

Fig. A1D. Relation between the mean response amplitude and the logarithm of the stimulus number

Table A3D Mean latency per stimulus level of the first (a) and the last(b) response

Stimulus levels	D_1		D_2		D_3		D_4	
	a	b	a	b	a	b	a	b
Latency	1.9	2.2	2.0	2.1	2.2	2.2	2.0	2.4

Table A4D Mean response duration per stimulus level of the first (a) and the last (b) response

Stimulus levels	D_1		D_2		D_3		D_4	
	a	b	a	b	a	b	a	b
Response duration	2.8	1.5	2.7	1.9	3.4	2.0	3.7	2.0

*Table A5D Mean pre-stimulus level per trial for the various stimulus levels in μMho's**

	1	2	3	4	5	6	7
D_1	11.97	12.31	12.50	12.54	12.63	12.61	12.64
D_2	10.14	10.51	10.64	10.59	10.60		
D_3	11.47	12.11	11.75	11.84	11.80	11.69	
D_4	10.93	11.53	11.47	11.49	11.48	11.45	

* Because of the wide dispersion only those values have been included for which $n = 10$.

Analyses

1. The effect of the stimulus levels on the habituation rate (HR).
   Because in several cases the value of HR attained 20, the non-parametric analysis of variance of Kruskal and Wallis was applied to the data of table A2D.
   $H = 8.64$; $p < 0.05$ (The difference between D_1 and D_2 is not significant; $H = 1.96$)
   The habituation rate increases significantly with longer stimulus duration, *i.e.* with an increase from 2.5 to 12.5 sec.

2. The effect of the stimulus levels on the amplitude of the first response.

Source of variance	Sum of squares	df	Mean square	F
Stimulus levels	1166.68	3	338.89	< 1.00
Ss within St. levels	17309.30	36	480.81	
Total	18475.98	39		

3. The effect of the stimulus levels on the latency of the first response.

Source of variance	Sum of squares	df	Mean square	F
Stimulus levels	0.40	3	0.13	< 1.00
Ss within St. levels	5.88	36	0.16	
	6.28	39		

4. The effect of the stimulus levels on the duration of the first response.

Source of variance	Sum of squares	df	Mean square	F
Stimulus levels	6.68	3	2.23	2.75 ($p < .10$)
Ss within St. levels	29.06	36	0.81	
Total	35.74	39		

Response duration tends to increase with increasing stimulus duration.

5. The linearity of the relation between the response amplitude and the logarithm of the stimulus number.
A total of 16 subjects was found to meet the criterion HR ≥ 8. For the stimulus numbers 1, 2, 4 and 8, that is, for 1, 2, 3 and 4 in the logarithmic scale, the mean amplitude was 38.3, 25.7, 14.9 and 7.0 respectively.
(N.B. These values are not the same as those in fig. A1D, where the number of measures per trial is not constant).

Source of variance	Sum of squares	df	Mean square	F
Stimulus numbers (T_r)	3460.55	3	1153.52	7.98 $p < .005$
Subjects (S)	4324.25	15	288.28	
$S \times T_r$	6502.13	45	144.49	
Total	14286.93	63		

L near component L = 3425.65 F = 23.71 $p < .005$
The function $y = -ax + b$, calculated by the method of least squares, was found to yield: $y = -6.54x + 29.78$.

6. The effect of the habituation process on the latency of the response as affected by the stimulus levels.

Source of variance	Sum of squares	df	Mean square	F
Stimulus levels (A)	.39	3	0.13	< 1.00
Ss within St. levels (B)	6.44	36	0.18	
Habituation (C)	1.03	1	1.03	8.58 $p < .01$
$A \times C$	0.36	3	0.12	1.00 n.s.
$B \times C$	4.38	36	0.12	
Total	12.60	79		

During the habituation process the response latency increases significantly.

7. The effect of the habituation process on the response duration as affected by the stimulus levels.

Source of variance	Sum of squares	df	Mean square	F
Stimulus levels (A)	6.91	3	2.30	3.90 $p<.025$
Ss within St. levels (B)	21.24	36	0.59	
Habituation (C)	32.39	1	32.39	58.89 $p<.005$
A × C	1.71	3	0.57	1.04 n.s.
B × C	19 72	36	0.55	
Total	81.87	79		

During the habituation process the response duration decreases significantly. The various stimulus levels show significant differences in this respect.

8. a) The relation between amplitude and latency of the first response. This correlation is not significant ($r = —.043$).
   b) The relation between amplitude and duration of the first response. This correlation is not significant ($r = .192$).

9. The relation between the amplitude of the first response and the habituation rate.
   The 'goodness-of-fit test' for normality applied to the habituation rate yielded: $X^2 = 16.4$ $p < .01$.
   In view of this result the rank correlation was computed as rho = .19 (n.s.)

10. The relation between $\triangle$ log C and the pre-stimulus level, log C.
    The correlation for the first response is not significant ($r = .180$).
    The correlation for the second response is not significant ($r = .059$).

11. The relation between the habituation rate and the onset value of log C. In view of the significant deviation from normality of the HR (see analysis 9) the rank correlation was computed as rho = .06 (n.s.).

12. The trend of the pre-stimulus level.
    In all cases there is an increase in the pre-stimulus level. This effect is apparently not influenced by the stimulus levels.

Summary

The HR is found to be affected only by the highest level of stimulus duration (12.5 sec), which is in accord with the findings of Sokolov (1963[b]). The amplitude of the response is found not to be affected by the duration of the stimulus, and neither is the response latency.

The hypothesis that there is a linear relation between the response amplitude ($\triangle$ log C) and the logarithm of the stimulus number has been confirmed. Yet another demonstration of the occurrence of habituation during stimulus repetition is furnished by the finding that the variance component 'stimulus numbers' in analysis 5 is significant. Habituation is found to be accompanied by increased response latency, but this effect is not significantly different for the various levels of stimulation.

Habituation also manifests itself in decreased response duration. In this case there are significant differences for the various levels of stimulation.

The low and non-significant correlations show that there is no appreciable connection between response amplitude, response duration and response latency.

The HR has been found to show little or no correlation with the amplitude of the first response.

Low, non-significant, correlations have been established between $\triangle$ log C and the pre-stimulus level log C, both for the first and the second response. No relation has been found to exist between the HR and the pre-stimulus level. During the experiment the pre-stimulus level increases.

A final point, not included in the general scheme of analysis, concerns the occurrence of 'terminal' OR's. Only in experimental condition D4 (stimulus duration 12.5 sec) can this effect be meaningfully studied. In 9 out of 10 cases this type of OR was found to occur; the corresponding HR was 8.5, significantly lower than for 'onset' OR's (16.2). This is in accord with the findings of Stern (1968).

5.3.2 Interstimulus interval

The four levels of the interstimulus interval, designated T_1, T_2, T_3 and T_4, were 5, 10, 20 and 40 sec.

Table A1T Mean response amplitude ($\triangle$ log C $\times$ 1000)

Data

Trials	Stimulus levels			
	T_1	T_2	T_3	T_4
1	31.3	32.2	23.6	24.3
2	5.1	7.9	8.9	14.3
3	1.9	1.8	5.3	9.3
4	2.9	1.8	2.8	8.9
5	0.9	1.1	2.5	8.4
6	0.5	0.2	3.7	3.7
7	2.8	3.0	1.3	5.3
8	0.5	1.1	0.9	5.1
9	0.4	0.1	0.6	4.5
10	0.0	0.5	1.1	7.1
11	0.0	1.2	0.7	5.4
12	0.0	0.3	2.1	6.1
13	0.3	0.1	0.0	2.2
14	0.5	0.1	0.1	2.8
15	0.1	0.0	0.6	2.8
16	0.1	0.0	0.7	2.9
17	0.0	0.0	0.2	1.3
18	0.0	0.0	0.8	1.9
19	0.0	0.0	0.8	0.4
20	0.0	0.0	0.3	1.9

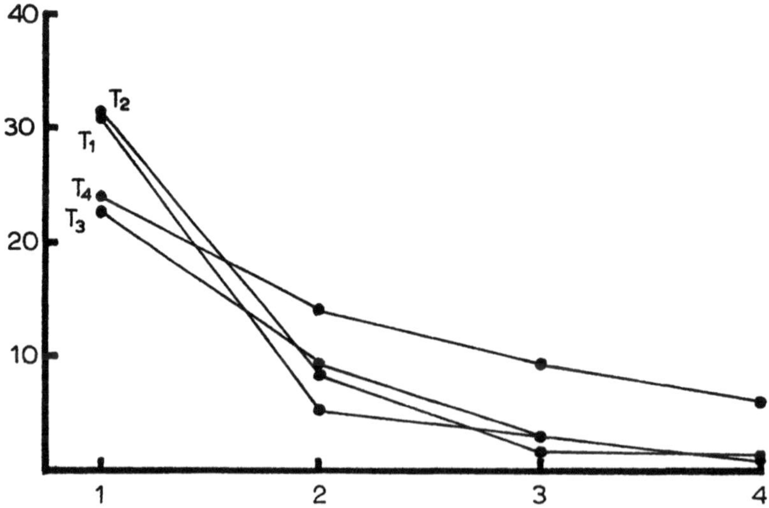

Fig. A1T. The relation between response amplitude and the logarithm of the stimulus number

Table A2T Mean value of the HR *per stimulus level*

Stimulus levels	T_1	T_2	T_3	T_4
Habituation rate	6.3	6.7	8.8	12.8

Table A3T Mean latency per stimulus level of the first (a), second (b) and last (c) response

Stimulus levels	T_1			T_2			T_3			T_4		
	a	b	c	a	b	c	a	b	c	a	b	c
Latency	1.4	1.4	1.6	1.4	1.5	1.7	2.0	2.1	2.1	1.4	1.4	1.7

Table A4T Mean response duration per stimulus level of the first (a), the second (b) and the last (c) response

Stimulus levels	T_1			T_2			T_3			T_4		
	a	b	c	a	b	c	a	b	c	a	b	c
Response duration	3.4	1.6	2.0	3.7	3.0	1.8	2.7	2.1	1.9	3.1	2.6	1.6

Table A5T Mean pre-stimulus level per trial and per stimulus level in μMho's (Only cell averages where n = 10 have been included)

	1	2	3	4	5	6	7	8	9	10
T_1	8.55	9.11	9.09	9.02	8.98	8.97	8.94	8.96	8.92	
T_2	8.91	8.94	8.92	8.94	8.97	8.87	8.94			
T_3	10.14	10.51	10.64	10.59	10.60					
T_4	8.69	8.86	8.90	8.90	8.95	9.22	8.96	8.96	9.20	9.09

Analyses

1. The effect of the stimulus levels on the habituation rate. Since the HR attains a value of twenty only once, a parametric analysis of variance was made.

Source of variance	Sum of squares	df	Mean square	F
Stimulus levels	266.6	3	88.7	2.91 $p < .05$
Ss within St. levels	1099.4	36	30.5	
Total	1366.0	39		

As the stimulus interval becomes longer, habituation proceeds more slowly.

2. The effect of the stimulus levels on the amplitude of the response. While in the other cases it is always the first response that is considered, this procedure is obviously impossible where the interstimulus-interval parameter is concerned. For this reason the second response is here considered. To determine whether a possible difference is to be attributed to sample fluctuations, the analysis is also carried out for the first response.

Amplitude first response

Source of variance	Sum of squares	df	Mean square	F
Stimulus levels	614.90	3	204.97	< 1.00
Ss within St. levels	14302.20	36	397.28	
Total	14917.10	39		

Amplitude second response

Source of variance	Sum of squares	df	Mean square	F
Stimulus levels	445.11	3	148.37	< 1.00
Ss within St. levels	5924.80	36	164.57	
Total	6369.91	39		

3. The effect of the stimulus levels on the response latency. The same remarks apply as under 2.

Latency first response

Source of variance	Sum of squares	df	Mean square	F
Stimulus levels	2.80	3	0.93	7.15 $p < .005$
Ss within St. levels	4.83	36	0.13	
Total	7.63	39		

Latency second response
Under condition T1 only 6 subjects gave a response. While amplitude and duration can in reason be assigned zero value, this is impossible for the response latency, since it correlates negatively with the amplitude. As a

result, the number of measures per subgroup was not the same, so that the non-parametric analysis of variance of Kruskal and Wallis was applied, $H = 15{,}51$; $p < .01$.

Significant differences exist among the latencies of both the first and the second response. These are unrelated to the interval parameter. Inspection of the data in table A3T will show that the effect is due to one extreme measure (T3).

4. The effect of the stimulus levels on the response duration. Again the same remarks apply as under 2.

Duration first response

Source of variance	Sum of squares	df	Mean square	F
Stimulus levels	8.84	3	2.95	1.21 $p > .25$
Ss within St. levels	87.78	36	2.44	
Total	96.62	39		

Duration second response

Source of variance	Sum of squares	df	Mean square	F
Stimulus levels	6.92	3	2.31	6.89 $p < .005$
Ss within St. levels	12.04	36	0.33	
Total	18.96	39		

The response duration decreases significantly with shorter stimulus intervals (see table A4T).

5. The linearity of the relation between the response amplitude and the logarithm of the stimulus number.
   There were 21 cases with HR ≥ 8. The logarithmic stimulus numbers 1, 2, 3 and 4 showed a mean response amplitude of 63.8, 26.3, 15.8 and 7.6 respectively.

Source of variance	Sum of squares	df	Mean square	F
Rank numbers (R)	8804.61	3	2934.87	27.08 $p < .005$
Subjects (Ss)	9365.24	20	468.26	
Ss × R	6503.14	60	108.39	
Total	24672.99	83		

The linear component L = 7637.34 F = 70.46 $p < .005$
The function $y = -ax + b$, determined by the method of least squares, was found to be: $y = -8.53 \times + 34.83$

6. The effect of the habituation process on the response latency as affected by the stimulus levels.

Source of variance	Sum of squares	df	Mean square	F
Stimulus levels (A)	4.47	3	1.49	7.10 $p < .005$
Ss within St. levels (B)	7.41	36	0.21	
Habituation (C)	1.35	1	1.35	16.88 $p < .005$
A × C	0.17	3	0.06	< 1.00
B × C	2.91	36	0.08	
Total	16.31	79		

During the habituation process the response latency increases significantly. While there are significant differences for the various stimulus levels, the effect is largely due to the very small increase at T3 (see table A3T).

7. The effect of the habituation process on the response duration as affected by the stimulus levels.

Source of variance	Sum of squares	df	Mean square	F
Stimulus levels (A)	5.84	3	1.95	< 1.00
Ss within St. levels (B)	82.88	36	2.30	
Habituation (C)	48.05	1	48.05	60.06 $p < .005$
A × C	3.90	3	1.30	1.63 n.s.
B × C	28.67	36	0.80	
Total	169.34	79		

During the habituation process the response duration decreases significantly.

8. The relation between
   a) amplitude and latency of the first response; $r = -.357$ $p < .025$
   b) amplitude and response duration of the first response; $r = .230$ (n.s.)

9. The relation between the amplitude of the first response and the habituation rate.
   The 'goodness-of-fit test' for normality produced the following result for the habituation rate: $X^2 = 26.8$ $p < .001$
   Because of this, a rank correlation was computed, rho $= 0.14$ (n.s.)
10. The relation between $\triangle$ log C and the pre-stimulus level log C.
    For the first response $r = .204$ (n.s.)
    For the second response $r = 0.285$ $p < .05$
11. The relation between the habituation rate and the onset value of log C.
    Since the HR deviated significantly from normality (see under 9) the rank correlation was computed as rho $= 0.31$ $p < .05$.
12. The trend of the pre-stimulus level.
    Again, an increase is observed in all cases. This effect is apparently not influenced by the stimulus levels.

Summary

The HR is found to increase systematically with increasing stimulus intervals. The effect is significant. This finding (decreasing habituation) is in accord with the results obtained by Geer (1966), who used longer intervals (20, 60 and 105 sec).

As regards the first response, the various subgroups show no significant differences for amplitude and response duration, but they do differ significantly with respect to response latency. The factor interstimulus interval has not been found to affect the amplitude of the second response. While the latencies of the second response differed significantly, this effect cannot in reason be attributed to the 'interval' parameter, since the same effect also occurs in the first response. The differences in duration of the second response are significant. Response duration decreases more quickly with shorter interstimulus intervals.

Again, the hypothesis that there is a linear relation between the response size ($\triangle$ log C) and the logarithm of the stimulus number has been confirmed. Habituation is found to be accompanied by a significant increase of the response latency and a significant decrease of the response duration. For the first response a significant negative correlation has been established between amplitude and latency. The correlation between amplitude and response duration is not significant; neither is the correlation between habituation rate and the amplitude of the first response.

Only for the second response are $\triangle$log C and log C found to be significantly correlated; however, the correlation is not high.

The onset value of log C and the habituation rate are likewise significantly correlated.

The pre-stimulus level increases during the experiment.

5.3.3 Interaction between duration and interstimulus interval

As stated before (5.1.3), a complementary experiment was carried out to study the possible interaction between the 'duration' and 'interval' parameters. The experiment provided data supplementary to those obtained under the conditions D_1 and D_3 with an interval of 20 sec (= T_3) (See 5.3.1). The new experimental conditions were again D_1 and D_3 but the interval was now 5 sec (= T_1). Before we discuss the interaction itself, we shall set out the new data (D_1 T_1 and D_3T_1).

Table A1DT Mean amplitude of the first response ($\triangle$ log C $\times$ 1000)

Stimulus levels	D_1T_1	D_3T_1
Amplitude	59.3	30.3

Table A2DT Mean habituation rate per stimulus level

Stimulus levels	D_1T_1	D_3T_1
Habituation rate	13.7	12.1

Table A3DT Mean latency per stimulus level of the first (a) and the last (b) response

Stimulus levels	D_1T_1		D_3T_1	
	a	b	a	b
Latency	1.2	1.3	1.7	2.0

Table A4DT Mean response duration per stimulus level of the first (a) and the last (b) response

Stimulus levels	D_1T_1		D_3T_1	
	a	b	a	b
Response duration	2.8	1.4	2.5	1.2

Analyses (general)

1. The effect of the stimulus levels on the habituation rate. Application of the test of Kruskal and Wallis produces $H = 2.366$ $p < .15$ (two-tailed).
2. The effect of the stimulus levels on the amplitude of the first response. The difference between the two samples was tested by means of the t-test; $t = 2.248$ $p < .05$ (two-tailed).
3. The effect of the stimulus levels on the latency of the first response. Application of the t-test produces $t = 3.417$ $p < .01$ (two-tailed).
4. The effect of the stimulus levels on the response duration. Application of the t-test produces $t = 0.886$ (n.s.)
5. The effect of the habituation process on response latency as affected by the stimulus levels.

Source of variance	Sum of squares	df	Mean square	F
Stimulus levels (A)	3.31	1	3.31	19.36 $p < .005$
Ss within St. levels (B)	3.09	18	0.17	
Habituation	0.38	1	0.38	4.22 $p < .10$
$A \times C$	0.27	1	0.27	3.00 (n.s.)
$B \times C$	1.56	18	0.09	
Total	8.61	39		

During the habituation process the latency tends to increase. The difference in increase between the two experimental conditions is significant (table A3DT).

6. The effect of the habituation process on response duration as affected by the stimulus levels.

Source of variance	Sum of squares	df	Mean square	F
Stimulus levels (A)	0.70	1	0.70	1.52 (n.s.)
Ss within St. levels (B)	8.29	18	0.46	
Habituation (c)	18.36	1	18.36	52.46 $p < .005$
A × C	0.03	1	0.03	< 1.00
B × C	6.28	18	0.35	
Total	33.66	39		

The response duration decreases significantly during the habituation process (table A4DT).

7. The relation between
   a) amplitude and latency of the first response; $r = -.269$ (n.s.)
   b) amplitude and response duration of the first response; $r = .513$ $p < .025$
8. The relation between the amplitude of the first response and the habituation rate.
   To this end, the rank correlation was computed as $\text{rho} = .57$ $p < .01$
9. The relation between the habituation rate and the onset value of log C $\text{rho} = .42$ $p < .05$

Interaction between duration and interstimulus intervals (continued)

The above results, combined with the data obtained under conditions D_1T_3 and D_3T_3 (see 5.3.1 under conditions D_1 and D_3) were used to answer the question whether the two factors exhibit interaction with regard to the habituation process. Habituation manifests itself most strongly on the first few trials of a stimulus sequence. It should be possible, therefore, to obtain a reasonable approximation of the degree of habituation by adopting as index the difference in response amplitude between, say, the first and the fifth response. However, the following chart showing the mean figures for the first responses will make it clear that absolute response decrease is not a very suitable measure.

		Duration	
		D_1	D_3
Interval	T_1	59.3	30.3
	T_3	24.7	21.4

(Since these are *first* responses, the differences between T_1 and T_3 must be regarded as sample fluctuations).

For this reason, the difference between the first and the fifth response, expressed as a percentage of the first response, was chosen as index.

This yielded the following figures:

		Duration	
		D_1	D_3
Interval	T_1	9.1%	20.1%
	T_3	32.4%	22.5%

Analysis of variance produced

Source of variance	Sum of squares	df	Mean square	F
Stimulus duration (D)	2.03	1	2.03	< 1.00
Stimulus interval (T)	1625.55	1	1625.55	2.53 (n.s.)
D × T	1071.18	1	1071.18	1.67 (n.s.)
Error	23096.06	36	641.56	
Total	25794.82	39		

The results show that neither stimulus duration nor stimulus interval has a significant effect on habituation (as a first response percentage). Nor is there significant interaction between these two terms.

A similar analysis of variance was applied to the mean latencies of the first five responses, as shown below.

		Duration	
		D_1	D_3
Interval	T_1	1.2	1.7
	T_3	2.0	2.1

Source of variance	Sum of squares	df	Mean square	F
Stimulus duration (D)	90.25	1	90.25	9.76 $p < .005$
Stimulus interval (T)	342.25	1	342.25	37.00 $p < .005$
D × T	42.25	1	42.25	4.57 $p < .05$
Error	333.00	36	9.25	
Total	807.75	39		

Both stimulus duration and intersitumulus interval are found to have a significant effect on response latency. The interaction between the two terms is likewise significant, *i.e.* the difference due to stimulus duration increases if the interstimulus interval is shorter. This interaction can be graphically represented as follows:

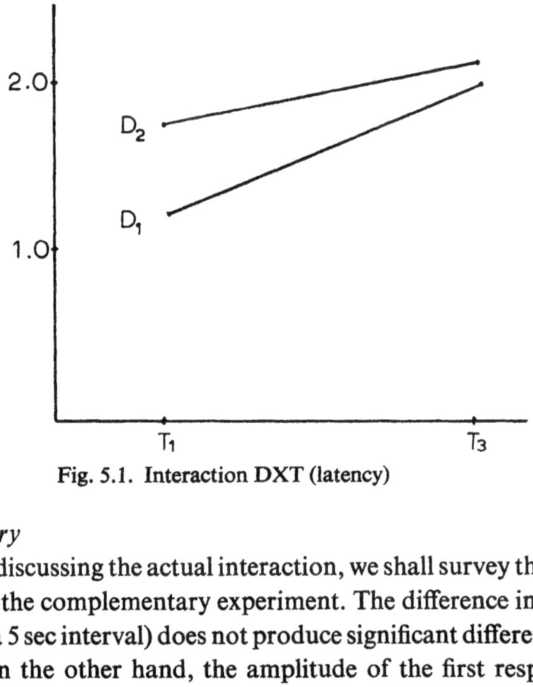

Fig. 5.1. Interaction DXT (latency)

Summary

Before discussing the actual interaction, we shall survey the findings from the data of the complementary experiment. The difference in stimulus duration (*i.e.* at a 5 sec interval) does not produce significant differences in habituation rate. On the other hand, the amplitude of the first response does show a significant effect due to stimulus duration. This also applies to the latency of the first response, but not to its duration. Habituation manifests itself in prolonged latency and decreased response duration. The increase in latency is strongly affected by stimulus duration.

While the correlation between amplitude and latency is not significant, that between amplitude and response duration *is*.

A fairly high significant correlation is found to exist between the amplitude of the first response and the habituation rate.

A similar correlation exists between the habituation rate and the onset value of log C. The interaction between stimulus duration and interstimulus interval is not significant as regards the degree of habituation expressed as a percentage of response decrease.

On the other hand, the interaction between the two stimulus parameters *was* significant as regards the mean latencies of the first five responses, as well as the variances due to two parameters separately.

5.3.4 Tone frequency

The different levels of this parameter have been designated F_1, F_2, F_3, F_4 and F_5 and are 500, 1000, 2000, 4000 and 8000 cps respectively.

Table A9F Mean response amplitude ($\triangle$ log C $\times$ 1000)

Data

	Stimulus levels				
Trials	F1	F2	F3	F4	F5
1	33.0	15.0	32.2	18.1	35.2
2	10.2	12.3	7.9	5.9	14.7
3	5.5	6.2	1.8	1.7	14.2
4	6.2	7.0	1.8	1.7	11.1
5	3.3	6.8	1.1	0.5	8.7
6	2.7	4.5	0.2	1.4	6.2
7	4.2	5.9	3.0	1.8	8.1
8	1.5	5.9	1.1	0.9	5.1
9	1.9	3.9	0.1	1.6	5.4
10	0.7	0.6	0.5	0.8	5.7
11	0.2	3.2	1.2	0.1	4.7
12	0.0	6.2	0.3	0.3	5.3
13	0.4	5.4	0.1	0.2	3.1
14	0.3	2.3	0.1	0.6	3.1
15	0.3	3.1	0.0	0.3	4.0
16	0.0	1.4	0.0	0.1	0.9
17	0.0	3.8	0.0	0.4	4.0
18	0.0	0.9	0.0	0.0	2.8
19	0.0	4.0	0.0	0.1	0.9
20	0.0	1.8	0.0	0.1	1.1

Table A2F Mean habituation rate per stimulus level

Stimulus levels	F_1	F_2	F_3	F_4	F_5
Habituation rate	9.1	12.4	6.7	9.8	12.5

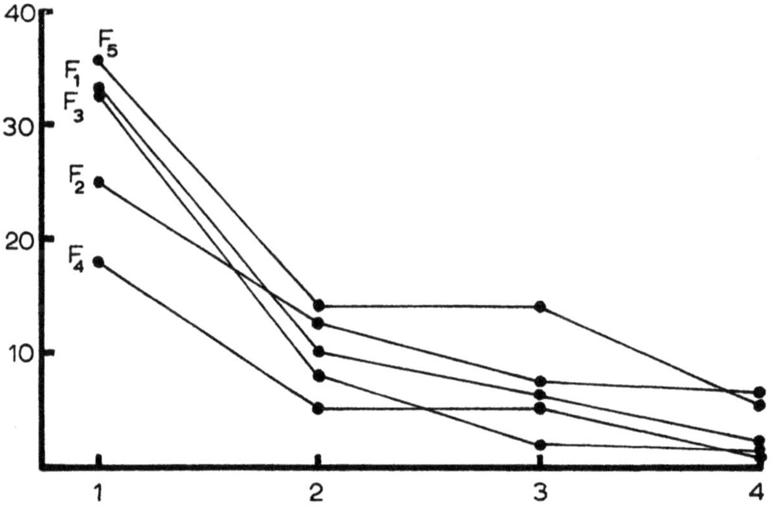

Fig. A1F. The relation between the response amplitude and the logarithm of the stimulus number

Table A3F Mean latency per stimulus level of the first (a) and the last (b) response

Stimulus levels	F1		F2		F3		F4		F5	
	a	b	a	b	a	b	a	b	a	b
Latency	1.9	2.0	2.0	2.2	1.3	1.4	1.9	2.2	1.8	2.1

Table A4F Mean response duration per stimulus level of the first (a) and the last (b) response

Stimulus levels	F1		F2		F3		F4		F5	
	a	b	a	b	a	b	a	b	a	b
Response duration	3.2	1.7	3.4	2.0	3.0	1.7	3.0	1.6	3.5	1.4

*Table A5F Mean pre-stimulus level per trial for the different stimulus levels in μMho's**

	1	2	3	4	5	6	7	8	9	10
F_1	6.24	6.64	6.71	6.73	6.80	6.75	6.80	6.74		
F_2	7.24	7.59	7.65	7.73	7.73	7.73	7.73	7.76	7.83	7.81
F_3	8.91	8.94	8.92	8.94	8.97	8.87	8.94			
F_4	9.00	9.16	9.19	9.17	9.20	9.21				
F_5	7.26	7.76	7.79	7.93	8.03	8.09	8.16	8.23	8.30	8.33

* Only those values have been included for which n= 10.

Analyses

1. The effect of the stimulus levels on the habituation rates. Because in several cases the HR attained a value of 20, the non-parametric analysis of variance of Kruskal and Wallis was applied.
   $H = 1.20$ (n.s.)

2. The effect of the stimulus levels on the amplitude of the first response

Source of variance	Sum of squares	df	Mean square	F
Stimulus levels	1990.40	4	497.60	1.21 (n.s.)
Ss within St. levels	18530.10	45	411.78	
Total	20520.50	49		

3. The effect of the stimulus levels on the latency of the first response

Source of variance	Sum of squares	df	Mean square	F
Stimulus levels	3.43	4	0.86	10.75 $p < .005$
Ss within St. levels	3.71	45	0.08	
Total	7.14	49		

As appears from these results, the latency of the response is significantly affected by the tone frequency. However, the data in table A3F show that the effect is not systematic. The deviating results obtained under conditions F_3 must probably be attributed to chance fluctuations.

4. The effect of the stimulus levels on the duration of the first response.

Source of variance	Sum of squares	df	Mean square	F
Stimulus levels	2.41	4	0.60	< 1.00
Ss within St. levels	49.19	45	1.09	
Total	51.60	49		

5. The linearity of the relation between the response amplitude and the logarithm of the stimulus number.
   The criterion HR ≥ 8 was met by 30 of the 50 subjects. The mean response amplitude for the logarithmic stimulus numbers 1, 2, 3 and 4 was 99.2, 38.0, 24.2 and 14.5 respectively.

Source of variance	Sum of squares	df	Mean square	F
Rank numbers (R)	14484.43	3	4828.14	43.05 $p < .005$
Subjects (Ss)	10875.74	29	375.03	
R × Ss	9754.82	87		
Total	35114.99	119		

The linear component L = 11961.74 F = 106.68 $p < .005$.
The function $y = -ax + b$, determined by the method of least squares, was found to be $y = -8.93x + 36.98$.

6. The effect of the habituation process on the latency of the response as affected by the stimulus levels.

Source of variance	Sum of squares	df	Mean square	F
Stimulus levels (A)	7.83	4	1.96	13.59 $p < .005$
Ss within St. levels (B)	6.48	45	0.14	
Habituation (C)	1.21	1	1.21	30.25 $p < .005$
A × C	1.77	4	0.44	11.00 $p < .005$
B × C	1.96	45	0.04	
Total	19.25	99		

During the habituation process the latency of the response increases significantly. The effect of the stimulus levels as well as the interaction between tone frequency and habituation is likewise significant.

7. The effect of the habituation process on the duration of the response as affected by the stimulus levels.

Source of variance	Sum of squares	df	Mean square	F
Stimulus levels (A)	2.19	4	0.55	< 1.00
Ss within St. levels (B)	46.58	45	1.04	
Habituation (C)	61.78	1	61.78	102.97 $p < .005$
A × C	2.22	4	0.56	< 1.00
B × C	26.93	45	0.60	
Total	139.70	99		

During the habituation process the duration of the response decreases significantly.

8. The relation between:
   a) amplitude and latency of the first response; $r = -.347$ $p < .01$
   b) amplitude and duration of the first response; $r = .190$ (n.s.)
9. The relation between the amplitude of the first response and the habituation rate.
   The 'goodness-of-fit test' for normality yielded for the habituation rate: $X^2 = 7.92$ $p > .10$. Although this p value is fairly high, a rank correlation was computed because the distribution of HR was found to be clearly bimodal; rho $= .35$ $p < .01$.
10. The relation between $\triangle$ log C and the pre-stimulus level log C.
    For the first response, $r = .120$ (n.s.)
    For the second response, $r = .113$ (n.s.)
11. The relation between the habituation rate and the onset value of log C. Because of the bimodal distribution of HR (see analysis 9) a rank correlation was computed.
    rho $= .24$ $p < .05$
12. The trend of the pre-stimulus level.
    Again, the pre-stimulus level is found to increase systematically for all the stimulus levels.

Summary

The tone frequency parameter does not affect the habituation rate. Nor does it affect the amplitude and the duration of the first response. On the other hand, the frequency does significantly affect the latency of the response, the effect being largely due to the low values of F3 (2000 cps). As stated before, this is probably a chance fluctuation; at least, the literature provides no indication to that effect. Again, the hypothesis concerning the linear relation between response amplitude and the logarithm of the stimulus number is confirmed.

The increase of the latency and the decrease of the response duration during the habituation process prove to be significant. The increase of the latency is affected by the tone frequency. The correlation between latency and amplitude is negative and significant; the correlation between response duration and amplitude is not significant.

A significant positive correlation exists between the amplitude of the first response and the habituation rate, and likewise between the onset value of log C and the habituation rate. The correlations between $\triangle$ log C and log C of the first and second responses are not significant. The pre-stimulus level increases significantly during the experiment.

5.3.5 Intensity

The various levels of stimulus intensity, designated I_1, I_2, I_3 and I_4 are 39, 59, 79 and 99 db respectively.

Table A11 Mean response amplitude ($\triangle$ log C $\times$ 1000)

	Stimulus levels			
Trials	I^1	I^2	I^3	I^4
1	30.2	32.2	63.3	93.7
2	7.2	7.9	22.3	42.7
3	1.5	1.8	12.2	35.9
4	6.2	1.8	18.2	26.2
5	4.3	1.1	11.6	25.7
6	1.2	0.2	15.1	13.6
7	0.6	3.0	9.9	16.7
8	0.5	1.1	6.6	19.7
9	2.2	0.1	1.9	15.7
10	0.1	0.5	4.9	16.3
11	1.5	1.2	0.7	7.3
12	0.6	0.3	4.1	7.4
13	0.0	0.1	2.9	2.6
14	0.4	0.1	5.0	4.4
15	0.2	0.0	2.7	2.9
16	0.0	0.0	4.8	4.0
17	0.0	0.0	1.0	4.4
18	0.1	0.0	3.3	3.7
19	0.0	0.0	2.3	1.3
20	0.0	0.0	0.1	2.2

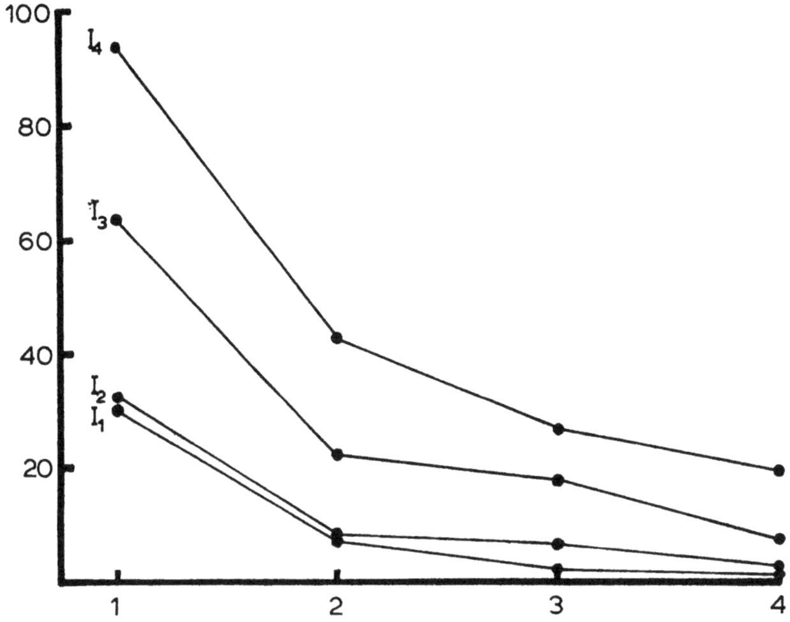

Fig. A11. The relation between response amplitude and the logarithm of the stimulus number

Table A2I Mean habituation rate per stimulus level

Stimulus levels	I_1	I_2	I_3	I_4
Habituation rate	8.9	6.7	11.9	18.2

Table A3I Mean latency per stimulus level of the first (a) and the last (b) response

Stimulus levels	I_1		I_2		I_3		I_4	
	a	b	a	b	a	b	a	b
Latency	1.9	1.9	1.3	1.5	1.7	2.0	1.5	1.8

Table A4I Mean response duration per stimulus level of the first (a) and the last (b) response

Stimulus levels	I_1		I_2		I_3		I_4	
	a	b	a	b	a	b	a	b
Response duration	3.0	1.5	3.1	1.9	3.7	1.7	4.6	1.8

*Table A5I Mean pre-stimulus level per trial for the various stimulus levels**

	1	2	3	4	5	6	7	8	9	10
I_1	7.14	7.61	7.62	7.56	7.63	7.63	7.58	7.54	7.52	7.50
I_2	8.66	9.16	9.21	9.32	9.36	9.37	9.36	9.37	9.39	
I_3	6.51	7.77	7.82	7.81	7.93	7.65	7.65	7.65	7.76	7.64
I_4	8.34	10.59	11.10	11.30	11.23	11.11	10.81	10.81	10.80	10.77

* Only those values have been included where $n = 10$

Analyses

1. The effect of the stimulus levels on the habituation rate. Because in several cases the value of the HR attained 20, the non-parametric analysis of variance of Kruskal and Wallis was applied to the data of table A2I. $H = 17.33$ $p < .001$
2. The effect of the stimulus levels on the amplitude of the first response.

Source of variance	Sum of squares	df	Mean square	F
Stimulus levels	27013.70	3	9004.57	3.71 $p < .025$
Ss within St. levels	87356.40	36	2426.57	
Total	114370.10	39		

The linear component $L = 24553.28$ $p < .005$
The response amplitude is apparently a linear function of the stimulus intensity.

3. The effect of the stimulus levels on the latency of the first response.

Source of variance	Sum of squares	df	Mean square	F
Stimulus levels	1.92	3	0.64	7.11 $p < .005$
Ss within St. levels	3.27	36	0.09	
Total	5.19	39		

The stimulus intensity has a significant effect on the latency of the first response. With the exception of I_2, the latency is found to decrease with increasing intensity.

4. The effect of the stimulus levels on the duration of the first response.

Source of variance	Sum of squares	df	Mean square	F
Stimulus levels	17.14	3	5.71	3.57 $p < .025$
Ss within St. levels	57.60	36	1.60	
Total	74.74	39		

The duration of the first response is an increasing function of the stimulus intensity.

5. The linearity of the relation between the response amplitude and the logarithm of the stimulus number. Since in this case both the amplitude of the first response and the habituation rate are significantly affected by the different stimulus levels and, moreover, a significant correlation is found to exist between the amplitude of the first response and the HR, the stimulus levels were included in the analysis of variance.
The analysis had to be restricted to the first three logarithmic stimulus numbers since only these yielded sufficient data. The number of subjects per stimulus level was eight. All of these met the criterion HR ≥ 4. The following chart lists the mean amplitude values.

	Stimulus number (log)		
	1	2	3
I_1	31.2	9.5	7.8
I_2	34.6	9.3	2.0
I_3	62.3	26.1	20.2
I_4	117.1	47.4	29.1

Source of variance	Sum of squares	df	Mean square	F
Stimulus levels (A)	34524.69	3	11508.23	6.12 $p < .005$
Ss within St. levels (B)	52664.92	28	1880.89	
Rank numbers (R)	31900.90	2	15950.45	23.25 $p < .005$
A × R	6893.76	6	1148.96	1.67 (n.s.)
B × R	38425.52	56	686.17	
Total	164409.79	95		

Since the interaction term A × R was found to be not significant, the linear component of the summated measures was computed.
$L = 28182.02 \quad F = 41.07\ p < .005$
The same coefficient of direction obtains for all the stimulus levels, since the interaction term A × R is not significant.
The value of this coefficient is —21.0. The value of b in the function $y = -ax + b$ was determined separately for each intensity. The functions for the various stimulus levels are as follows,
$I_1 \quad y = -21.0x + 39.6$
$I_2 \quad y = -21.0x + 47.9$
$I_3 \quad y = -21.0x + 78.3$
$I_4 \quad y = -21.0x + 152.5$

6. The effect of the habituation process on the latency of the response as affected by the stimulus levels.

Source of variance	Sum of squares	df	Mean square	F
Stimulus levels (A)	2.99	3	3.00	14.28 $p < .005$
Ss within St. levels (B)	7.41	36	0.21	
Habituation (C)	1.06	1	1.06	13.25 $p < .005$
A × C	0.21	3	0.07	< 1.00
B × C	2.95	36	0.08	
Total	14.62	79		

During the habituation process the latency increases significantly. This effect is significantly affected by the stimulus levels.

7. The effect of the habituation process on the duration of the response as affected by the stimulus levels.

Source of variance	Sum of squares	df	Mean square	F
Stimulus levels (A)	9.81	3	3.27	2.09 (n.s.)
Ss within St. levels (B)	56.29	36	1.56	
Habituation (C)	70.69	1	70.69	82.20 $p < .005$
A × C	8.08	3	2.69	3.13 $p < .10$
B × C	31.07	36	0.86	
Total	175.94	79		

During the habituation process the duration of the response decreases significantly.

8. The relation between
   a) amplitude and latency of the first response: $r = -.167$ (n.s.)
   b) amplitude and duration of the first response: $r = .493$ $p < .005$.
9. The relation between the amplitude of the first response and the habituation rate.
   The 'goodness-of-fit test' for normality yielded for the habituation rate:
   $X^2 = 11.6$ $p < .05$
   The rank correlation was computed as rho $= .49$ $p < .01$
10. The relation between Δ log C and the pre-stimulus level, log C.
    For the first response, $r = .133$ (n.s.)
    For the second response, $r = .360$ $p < .025$
11. The relation between the habituation rate and the onset value of log C.
    In view of the result of analysis 9, a rank correlation was computed; rho $= .27$ $p < .05$
12. The trend of the pre-stimulus level.
    There is an increase in the pre-stimulus level in all cases. This increase becomes more pronounced with increasing stimulus intensity.
    Percentage expression of the differences yields the following results:

Stimulus level	I_1	I_2	I_3	I_4
Change of pre-stimulus level in %	5.6	8.4	17.4	29.1

The effect, *i.e.* the increase of the percentage with increasing intensity, was significant:
$X^2 = 22.28$ $p < .001$

Summary

The habituation rate increases systematically with increasing stimulus intensity; this effect is significant.

A similar result is obtained for the amplitude of the first response, the relation between amplitude and intensity being linear. This provides confirmation for the findings of Leavy and Geer (1967) and of Uno and Grings (1965). First response latency and response duration are significantly affected by stimulus intensity. In general, latency decreases with increasing stimulus intensity, whereas response duration increases systematically.

A linear relation exists between the response amplitude and the logarithm of the stimulus number (first four trials). The interaction between the factor 'stimulus numbers' and 'stimulus intensity' is not significant, or to put it differently, the linear functions for the different intensities show the same coefficient of direction. Habituation produces longer latencies; the increase is significantly affected by stimulus intensity.

The decrease in response duration is also significant; it is not significantly affected by stimulus intensity.

No significant correlation exists between response latency and the amplitude of the first response; on the other hand, there *is* a (positive) correlation between amplitude and response duration.

The correlation between habituation rate and first response amplitude is positive and significant. While there is no significant correlation between $\triangle$ log C and log C for the first response, there *is* for the second response.

A significant positive correlation is exhibited by the habituation rate and the onset value of log C. The prestimulus level increases systematically. This increase becomes systematically more pronounced with increasing stimulus intensity.

5.3.6 General summary

In general, the habituation rate is found to increase (= the habituation process proceeds more slowly) with increasing stimulus duration, intensity and interval. Tone frequency shows no effect. As regards duration and intensity of the stimulations, this finding is in accord with Sokolov (1963), while the results for the stimulus interval are in agreement with Geer (1966) (see Ch 3.2).

The amplitude of the first response and the response duration are influenced only by the stimulus intensity. Intensity, tone frequency and interstimulus interval affect the response latency. The relation between stimulus intensity and response latency is of a general nature and holds for a great many response systems.

As has been shown before (see the summary of 5.3.2), the differences in latency occurring upon variation of the interval factor cannot be attributed to the effect of the stimulus interval, but are due to sample fluctuation. Latency is not systematically affected by tone frequency; only the 2000 cps tones produced shorter latencies. It would appear that no great importance must be attached to this finding.

The interaction between stimulus duration and stimulus interval is significant only in the case of response latency. That is to say, the difference in latency due to stimulus duration increases with decreasing stimulus intervals.

Under all stimulus conditions a linear relation is found to exist between $\triangle$ log C and the logarithm of the stimulus number. This is in agreement with the views of Montagu and Coles (1966) (see Ch 3.2.1). It follows that the curve representing the relation between $\triangle$ log C and the stimulus number is not an exponential function.

Habituation is always accompanied by increased response latency and decreased response duration. In some cases these effects are influenced by the stimulus levels. Increased latency and decreased response duration upon stimulus repetition have also been reported by Koepke and Pribram (1966).

The correlations between amplitude and latency as well as between amplitude and response duration, both for the first response, are given below.

Stimulus parameter	*Correlation Ra-Lt*	*Correlation Ra-Rd*
Stimulus duration	$r = -.043$ (n.s.)	$r = .192$ (n.s.)
Stimulus interval	$r = -.357$ $p < .025$	$r = .230$ (n.s.)
Tone frequency	$r = -.347$ $p < .01$	$r = .190$ (n.s.)
Stimulus intensity	$r = -.167$ (n.s.)	$r = .493$ $p < .005$

The correlations between amplitude and latency are all negative and sometimes significant. This implies that a larger response will in general show a shorter latency. The correlations between amplitude and response duration are all positive but mostly not significant. Apparently, the form of the response wave is not entirely dependent on the amplitude. Put another way, a response wave may assume different forms while the amplitude is the same. This applies to a far smaller extent when the stimulus intensity is manipulated as independent variable.

For the variables stimulus intensity and tone frequency the habituation rate is found to correlate with the amplitude of the first response (rho $=$ .49, $p < .01$ and rho $= .35$, $p < .01$ respectively).

Stimulus intensity is thus found to dominate to a marked extent over the other stimulus properties in its effect on the various response variables.

The correlations between $\triangle$ log C and log C are given below.

	First response	*Second response*
Stimulus duration	r = .180 (n.s.)	r = .059 (n.s.)
Interstimulus interval	r = .204 (n.s.)	r = .285 $p < .05$
Tone frequency	r = .120 (n.s.)	r = .113 (n.s.)
Stimulus intensity	r = .133 (n.s.)	r = .360 $p < .025$

In the first response $\triangle$ log C is therefore independent of log C. Remarkably, the second response exhibits some significant correlations. This shows that the value of $\triangle$ log C is not always quite so independent of the pre-stimulus level as is generally assumed.

The correlations between the onset value of log C and the habituation rate are as follows:

Stimulus duration	rho = .06 (n.s.)
Interstimulus interval	rho = .31 $p < .05$
Tone frequency	rho = .24 $p < .05$
Stimulus intensity	rho = .27 $p < .05$

These correlations may indicate that there is a certain relation between arousal level and habituation rate. In other words, there is a tendency for the habituation process to proceed more slowly at higher arousal levels. Now, spontaneous activity is also used as an index of the arousal level. For this reason the correlations with the spontaneous activity over a period of three minutes prior to the start of the experiment were also determined. This was done whenever the particular stimulus parameter showed a significant effect on the habituation rate.

Correlation spontaneous activity – habituation rate:

Stimulus duration	D1	rho = .00
	D2	rho = .66 $p < .05$
	D3	rho = .50 (n.s.)
	D4	rho = .86 $p < .01$
Interstimulus interval	T1	rho = .17 (n.s.)
	T2	rho = .21 (n.s.)
	T3	rho = .69 $p < .05$
	T4	rho = .37 (n.s.)
Tone frequency		r = .186 (n.s.)

Stimulus intensity	I1	rho = .37 (n.s.)
	I2	rho = —.49 (n.s.)
	I3	rho = .24 (n.s.)
	I4	rho = .75 $p < .01$

Aside from the correlation under I2, all the correlations are positive and sometimes fairly high. This may be regarded as confirmation of the above-mentioned tendency for the habituation process to proceed more slowly at higher arousal levels.

The relation observed between spontaneous activity and habituation rate is furthermore in accord with the findings of Johnson (1963), Koepke and Pribram (1966) and of Lader and Wing (1964).

Important in this connection is also the finding that under all stimulus conditions the pre-stimulus level (absolute conductance) increases systematically during the experiment. Lader and Wing (1964) found that an increase in conductance level is characteristic of anxious individuals. They also found that anxiety delays the habituation process. These various findings could indicate that the experimental situation affected the subjects emotionally.

Aside from the above increase in conductance level there is also an increase due to stimulus intensity, since the increase in conductance level is found to increase systematically with increasing stimulus intensity.

Finally, it should be mentioned that if the stimulus is of relatively long duration (12.5 sec), so-called terminal OR's occur, which habituate much more quickly (about twice as rapidly) than the OR to the onset of the stimulus. This confirms the findings of Stern (1968) (see Ch 1.7 and the summary of 5.3.1).

6 DISHABITUATION DUE TO STIMULUS CHANGE WITHIN ONE DIMENSION

Following the habituation process, that is, after three successive stimulations had produced no response, one stimulus property was changed, while all the other stimulus characteristics remained the same. This altered stimulus was now repeated regularly until habituation again occurred. The central question here is in what way dishabituation manifests itself. In view of the varying nature of the dishabituation phenomena no general scheme for data analysis will be presented. Each stimulus parameter will be treated separately.

The changes in stimulation are set out below. Column I gives the value of the particular parameter before the change. Column II gives the changed stimulus.

Table 6.1

Stimulus factor	I	II
Duration (interstimulus interval 20 sec)	0.1 sec	0.5 sec
	0.5 sec	0.1 sec
	2.5 sec	12.5 sec
	12.5 sec	2.5 sec
Duration (interstimulus interval 5 sec)	0.1 sec	2.5 sec
	0.5 sec	12.5 sec
Interstimulus interval	5 sec	10 sec
	10 sec	5 sec
Tone frequency	500 cps	1000 cps
	500 cps	2000 cps
	500 cps	4000 cps
	500 cps	8000 cps
	1000 cps	500 cps
	2000 cps	500 cps
	4000 cps	500 cps
	8000 cps	500 cps

Stimulus factor	I	II
Intensity	39 db	59 db
	39 db	79 db
	39 db	99 db
	59 db	39 db
	79 db	39 db
	99 db	39 db

Under each stimulus condition 10 observations were made. Successively, the effects of changes in stimulus duration, interstimulus interval, tone frequency and stimulus intensity will be discussed. In all these cases the effect of the so-called intersession habituation will be studied as well. This phenomenon – mentioned in Ch 5.2 ('potentiation of habituation') – manifests itself in decreased responsivity upon repetition of a stimulus sequence after initial habituation.

While the quantitative changes in one stimulus aspect somewhat impair exact repetition of the sequence, the modifications are after all fairly minor ones. It therefore seems natural to assume that the decrease in responsivity will be generalized to the modified stimulus, which still has many properties in common with the original stimulus. In the following pages the term intersession habituation will be used to refer to the phenomenon of generalized intersession habituation.

6.1 DISHABITUATION DUE TO MODIFICATION OF STIMULUS DURATION

6.1.1 Modifications in the duration of the stimuli

Table 6.2

Interval	20 sec				5 sec	
Original duration	0.1 sec	0.5 sec	2.5 sec	12.5 sec	0.1 sec	2.5 sec
Modified duration	0.5 sec	0.1 sec	12.5 sec	2.5 sec	0.5 sec	12.5 sec

For each condition of stimulus modification again 10 subjects were used, that is, 60 subjects in all. The data are presented in the following tables.

Table 6.3 Mean amplitude (Δ log C $\times$ 1000) after stimulus modification

Change in duration	I 0.1 → 0.5 sec	II 0.5 → 0.1 sec	III 2.5 → 12.5 sec	IV 12.5 → 2.5 sec
Interval 20 sec	14.8 (n = 10)	8.9 (n = 8)	1.0 (n = 3)	9.5 (n = 10)
Interval 5 sec	24.0 (n = 10)		16.5 (n = 8)	

n = number of subjects giving a response after stimulus modification

Table 6.4 Mean response duration after stimulus modification

Change in duration	I 0.1 → 0.5 sec	II 0.5 → 01 sec	III 2.5 → 12.5 sec	IV 12.5 → 2.5 sec
Interval 20 sec	2.8 sec	1.9 sec	2.7 sec	1.8 sec
Interval 5 sec	2.1 sec		2.1 sec	

Table 6.5 Mean response latency after stimulus modification

Change in duration	I 0.1 → 0.5 sec	II 0.5 → 0.1 sec	III 2.5 → 12.5 sec	IV 12.5 → 2.5 sec
Interval 20 sec	2.0 sec	2.2 sec	4.9 sec	4.1 sec
Interval 5 sec	1.3 sec		5.2 sec	

Table 6.6 Mean habituation rate after stimulus modification

Change in duration	I 0.1 → 0.5 sec	II 0.5 → 0.1 sec	III 2.5 → 12.5 sec	IV 12.5 → 2.5 sec
Interval 20 sec	5.5	3.6	5.5	5.5
Interval 5 sec	10.3		8.8	

Table 6.7 Mean values (for all subjects) of the first response (A) and the last response (B) prior to stimulus modification, and of the first response (C) after stimulus modification

	A	B	C
Amplitude	36.0	5.8	14.2
Response duration	3.0	1.6	2.2

Table 6.8 Mean habituation rate (for all subjects) before (A) and after (B) stimulus modification

	A	B
Habituation rate	13.0	6.7

6.1.2 Problem specifications and analyses

Generally speaking, dishabituation should manifest itself in increased response amplitude and duration and decreased response latency. Of the total of 60 subjects 49 were found to respond after stimulus modification. The majority of these, 34 subjects, had attained complete habituation in the preceding sequence, while of the remaining subjects 14 clearly made a larger response after stimulus modification. Dishabituation therefore occurred in 80% of the subjects (n = 48).

We shall now attempt to answer a number of specific questions by analysis of the data.

1. Is the difference between the mean amplitude values of the (last) response before and the first response after stimulus modification significant?
   For the 48 subjects showing dishabituation the mean amplitude of the (last) response was 5.8 as against 14.2 after stimulus modification. Application of the t-test for related measures yielded $t = 4.15$ $p < .005$.
2. A similar question was asked with respect to response duration. The mean values of the response duration before and after stimulus modification were 1.6 and 2.2 respectively. The difference was significant: $t = 2.99$ $p < .005$.*
3. Does the response amplitude exhibit intersession habituation?
   Intersession habituation should manifest itself in a decrease in response amplitude upon comparison of the first response before and the first response after dishabituation. Naturally, only the 48 cases mentioned above will be considered since intersession habituation presupposes the occurrence of dishabituation.

* No attempt was made to study the effect of the nature of the stimulus modification on the dishabituation response. Prior to dishabituation the subgroups were not homogeneous as regards, for instance, the amplitude of the first response and the habituation rate.

The mean values of the two first response amplitudes were 36.0 and 14.2 respectively. This difference is significant: $t = 7.11$ $p < .005$.

4. A similar question was asked with regard to response duration. The values were 3.0 and 2.2 respectively. This difference is significant: $t = 3.90$ $p < .005$.
5. Intersession habituation should also manifest itself in a decreased habituation rate after dishabituation. Prior to dishabituation the mean HR was 13.0, after dishabituation 6.7. The Wilcoxon test for paired observations yielded: $T = 19.5$, $z = 5.55$ $p < .001$.
6. What changes does modification of the stimulus duration produce in the response latency? For a better understanding of the data, these are presented together with values for the preceding habituation (Ch 5.3.1 and 5.3.3).

Table 6.9 A survey of response latencies

Interval	Condition	a	c	c	Difference c — b[2]
20″	III + IV[1]	1.5	1.8	4.3	$T = 1$; $p < .005$
5″	III (2.5 → 12.5 sec)	1.7	2.0	5.2	$T = 0$; $p < .005$
20″	I (0.1 → 0.5 sec)	1.4	1.6	2.0	$T = 31$; $p < .01$[3] (rows 20″ I and 20″ II combined)
20″	II (0.5 → 0.1 sec)	1.5	1.7	2.2	
5″	I (0.1 → 0.5 sec)	1.2	1.3	1.3	

a) = Lt of the first response of the preceding habituation sequence.
b) = Lt of the last response of the preceding habituation sequence.
c) = Lt of the first response after stimulus modification (dishabituation).
1) Since at the 20 sec interval under cond. III only 3 subjects responded, the data under III and IV have been combined in this case.
2) The Wilcoxon test has been applied.
3) The two groups were combined because the difference between conds. I and II was not significant.

The question now arises whether the change in stimulus duration can be shown to produce dishabituation. Dishabituation in itself causes shorter latencies compared with the last response before dishabituation. Because of intersession habituation, however, the Lt of the first response after dishabituation will still exceed the Lt of the first response of the preceding habituation sequence. A reasonable estimate of the Lt after dishabituation is the mean of the first and the last response of the preceding habituation sequence.

If, however, the stimulus duration is modified, this estimated Lt must be augmented by the shortest stimulus duration. This can be demonstrated as follows. If stimulus duration a > stimulus duration b, the stimulus modification, either in the change-over from a→b or from b→a, will produce no effect until at least b seconds have elapsed since the start of stimulation.

It follows that if a response is made to the change in stimulus duration, the Lt actually measured must *at least* equal the estimated Lt augmented by the shortest stimulus duration. This point will now be ascertained for the four different cases.

Conditions III and IV (interval 20 sec)
The estimated Lt is (1.5 + 1.8) / 2 = 1.7, the shortest stimulus duration 2.5, total 4.2 sec. The obtained value is 4,3 sec.

Condition III (interval 5 sec)
The estimated Lt is (1.7 + 2.0) / 2 = 1.9, the shortest stimulus duration is 2.5, total 4.4 sec. The obtained value is 5.2 sec.

Conditions I and II (interval 20 sec)
The estimated Lt is (1.4 + 1.6 + 1.5 + 1.7) / 4 = 1.6, the shortest stimulus duration 0.1, total 1.7 sec.
The obtained value is 2.1 sec.

Condition I (interval 5 sec)
The differences are too small to allow conclusions.

Under most conditions the requirement has been met that the actual Lt should at least equal the estimated Lt augmented with the shortest stimulus duration. The conclusion is justified that, upon modification of the stimulus duration, the change actually causes dishabituation.

7. Finally, the question may be asked whether a relation exists between dishabituation and the subject's reported perception or non-perception of the change in stimulus duration. Unfortunately, no verbal reports were available of all the subjects. Of 38 subjects showing dishabituation 37 were found to have perceived the change in stimulation. Over against this must be set the fact that 10 subjects who showed no dishabituation all reported having perceived the stimulus change. The relation therefore is not entirely clear.

Summary

In 80% of all cases changes in stimulus duration subsequent to habituation have been found to cause dishabituation. This dishabituation manifests itself in a significant increase in both amplitude and response duration and is apparently accompanied by perception of the stimulus change. This latter finding cannot be reversed, however!

The phenomenon of intersession habituation – which Thompson and Spencer (1966) termed potentiation of habituation – is clearly demonstrated by the significant decrease in response amplitude after dishabituation, as compared with the amplitude of the first response prior to dishabituation. The same finding has been obtained for response duration (generalization of intersession habituation).

Attainment of renewed habituation after dishabituation requires only half the original number of trials. From the increase in latencies it can be inferred that in general dishabituation is caused by the change in stimulus duration. This is in accord with the findings of Koepke and Pribram (1966).

6.2 DISHABITUATION DUE TO MODIFICATION OF THE INTERSTIMULUS INTERVAL

Only a small-scale experiment has been conducted on this form of dishabituation. The first group (n = 10), which initially received a tone of 2000 cps, 59 db and 0.5 sec duration at 5 sec intervals, was upon habituation presented with the same tone, but now at 10 sec intervals, until again complete habituation occurred (group A). For the second group (n = 10) the situation was reversed, *i.e.* the initial 10 sec interval was upon habituation changed to 5 sec (group B).

After interval modification only 2 subjects in group B were found to make a response exceeding the last response prior to interval modification both as regards amplitude and response duration; in one case the latency was also shortened. This means that shortening of the interval probably does not produce dishabituation. Thr situation is a little more complicated with group A. First, after lengthening of the interval the actual stimulus may evoke a response but, secondly, a response may occur at the moment (after 5 sec) when the stimulus could be expected but did not actually occur.

We shall first consider the first type of response, the response to the actual stimulus. Of 10 subjects 4 were found to show a response amplitude exceeding that of the last response before modification of the interval. Two of them also showed increased response duration, while the latency became shorter in only one case. In all four cases the habituation rate had become lower after modification of the interval than it had been before, the mean values being 9.0 and 5.8 respectively.

The second type of response – to the absence of the stimulus – was not obtained. True, in three cases a response occurred, but the latencies were too small to allow the responses to be regarded as due to dishabituation. All the subjects who made a dishabituation response to the actual stimulation (6 in all) had perceived the change in interstimulus interval. However, in 8 other cases where no dishabituation response was made the change was perceived as well. These findings indicate than dishabituation as a result of interval change does not occur invariably.

6.3 DISHABITUATION DUE TO CHANGES IN TONE FREQUENCY

In two experiments the data of 80 subjects on this score were obtained.

The first group (A), consisting of 40 subjects, received a tone of 500 cps, 56 db, duration 0.5 sec, repeated every 10 sec. After habituation or 20 stimulations the tone frequency was changed. For the four different groups, each consisting of 10 subjects, the new frequency, of 1000 cps, 2000 cps, 4000 cps or 8000 cps, was corrected for subjective loudness. The data are summarized in table 6.10 and a section of table 6.12.

The second group (B), likewise consisting of 40 subjects, was at once subdivided into four subgroups of 10 subjects each. These subjects received a tone of either 1000 cps (60 db), or 2000 cps (59 db), or 4000 cps (54 db) or 8000 cps (65 db). After habituation or 20 stimulations all the subgroups received a tone of 500 cps (56 db), while all other conditions remained unchanged. In both cases the sequence was continued after the stimulus change until habituation was complete, up to a maximum of 20 stimulations. The data are presented in table 6.11 and in a section of table 6.12.

Table 6.12 Mean habituation rate prior to (a) and after (b) stimulus change

	a	b	a	b	a	b	a	b
Group A	500 cps	1000 cps	500 cps	2000 cps	500 cps	4000 cps	500 cps	8000 cps
	9.1	4.0	11.5	5.5	9.9	6.2	10.2	12.0
Group B	12.2	6.0	9.0	4.3	9.8	6.9	12.5	6.1
	1000 cps	500 cps	2000 cps	500 cps	4000 cps	500 cps	8000 cps	500 cps

Table 6.10 (group A)

	I	II	III	I	II	III	I	II	III	I	II	III
Stimulus	500 cps	500 cps	1000 cps	500 cps	500 cps	2000 cps	500 cps	500 cps	4000 cps	500 cps	500 cps	8000 cps
Ampl.*	36.0	1.5	24.1	25.4	1.3	15.3	23.5	2.9	13.2	24.1	6.7	18.1
Resp. duration	3.2	1.7	2.6	3.1	1.9	2.7	3.4	1.8	2.1	2.7	1.8	2.5
Latency	1.9	2.0	1.9	1.9	2.2	2.0	1.9	2.0	2.2	1,7	1.9	1.9

* $\triangle \log C \times 1000$
I = mean first response before stimulus change
II = mean last response before stimulus change
III = mean first response after stimulus change

Table 6.11 (group B)

	I	II	III	I	II	III	I	II	III	I	II	III
Stimulus	1000 cps	1000 cps	500 cps	2000 cps	2000 cps	500 cps	4000 cps	4000 cps	500 cps	8000 cps	8000 cps	500 cps
Ampl.*	25.0	5.0	13.8	29.9	4.3	23.5	18.1	1.3	12.0	35.2	4.0	13.4
Resp. duration	3.4	2.0	2.4	3.0	1.7	2.4	3.0	1.6	2.3	3.5	1.4	2.2
Latency	2.0	2.2	2.1	1.3	1.4	1.3	1.9	2.2	1.9	1.8	2.2	1.9

* $\triangle \log C \times 1000$
I = mean first response before stimulus change
II = mean last response before stimulus change
III = mean first response after stimulus change

Data processing and analysis

The first question studied was whether dishabituation occurred as a result of stimulus change. To this end, the number of cases was determined, both for group A and for group B, in which the amplitude of the first response after stimulus modification exceeded that of the last response before the stimulus change or, alternatively, was larger than zero if habituation had already been complete. In group A 36 of the 40 cases showed dishabituation. In group B 36 of the 40 cases showed dishabituation.

Problems and analyses

1. To what extent is the difference in amplitude between the last response before stimulus change and the first response after stimulus change significant?
   For the total group (group A + group B) this difference was tested by means of the t-test. The mean values were 3.5 and 17.1 respectively; $t = 7.84$ $p < .005$.
2. Is the difference in response duration before and after stimulus change significant (group A + group B)? The mean values were 1.7 and 2.4 respectively; $t = 7.18$ $p < .005$.
3. Is the difference in latency before and after stimulus change significant? From one of the previous analyses it had been found that the latency was significantly affected by the tone frequency. Inspection of the tables 6.10 and 6.11 shows that this effect is largely due to group B. Moreover, group B exhibits a systematic decrease in latency upon stimulus change whereas group A does not. The problem was therefore dealt with separately for the two groups.
   Group A: Here only the t-test was applied. The mean values were 2.0 and 2.0 $t = 0.20$ (n.s.)
   Group B: In this case an analysis of variance for repeated measures was applied:

Source of variance	Sum of squares	df	Mean square	F
Stimulus distance (Sdi)	7.84	3	2.61	18.64 $p < .01$
Ss within St. distances (Ss)	4.99	36	0.14	
Stimulus change (Sch)	0.47	1	0.47	5.88 $p < .025$
Sdi × Sch	0.12	3	0.04	< 1.00
Ss × Sch	2.87	36	0.08	
Total	16.29	79		

The change in tone frequency causes significant shortening of the latency. This effect is significantly influenced by the degree of change. Table 6.11 (change-over from II to III) shows that the shortening is greatest with the larger stimulus distances (4000, and 8000 cps → 500 cps).

Intersession habituation

4. Does the response amplitude exhibit intersession habituation?
   To this end, the difference between the first response before and the first response after stimulus change was tested for the total group (group A + group B). The mean values were 27.7 and 17.1 respectively; $t = 8.12$ $p < .005$.
5. A similar question was asked with regard to response duration.
   The mean values were 3.2 and 2.4 respectively. This difference proved to be significant ($t = 6.02$; $p < .005$).
6. The question as to whether the latencies exhibited intersession habituation was answered separately for the two groups A and B.
   Group A The mean values were 1.9 and 2.0. This difference was significant ($t = 2.61$; $p < .025$).
   Group B Since the latencies are here significantly influenced by the nature of the stimulus change, an analysis of variance was performed.

Source of variance	Sum of squares	df	Mean square	F
Tone frequency (T)	646.45	3	215.48	14.25 $p < .005$
Ss within T's (Ss)	544.10	36	15.11	
Intersession habituation (I)	12.80	1	12.80	4.39 $p < .05$
T × I	9.30	3	3.1	1.06 (n.s.)
Ss × I	104.90	36	2.91	
Total	1317.55	79		

The latency of the first response after stimulus change is significantly longer than that of the first response of the original sequence (before habituation). This means that intersession habituation has occurred. The degree of stimulus change (distance in tone frequency) very clearly affects this phenomenon. Table 6.11 (change-over from I to III) shows that this latter effect is not systematic, but occurs only with the largest and the smallest stimulus distances.

7. Does the habituation rate exhibit intersession habituation?

This point was determined for the total group (group A + group B) by testing the difference by means of the Wilcoxon test.
The mean values were 10.6 and 6.4.
$T = 408.5$ $z = 5.27$ $p < .0001$.

8. Finally, the effect of the stimulus change on the mean conductance level was determined. In the last chapter (5.3.4) we had already found that this level increases during the habituation process. Dishabituation, it now appears, produces no change in this respect. On comparing the pre-stimulus level of the last response before stimulus change with that of the *second* response after stimulus change, we find the mean values of log C to be 0.856 and 0.865 (No error of transposition is involved!).
This increase was significant ($F = 12.19$; $p < .005$).

The effect of the stimulus distance and the direction of change
As has already appeared from the description of the experiment, the size of the dishabituation effect can be studied as a function of the stimulus distance. For each range this can be done in both directions, from low to high (group A) and from high to low (group B). From the data of group A a dishabituation gradient can be constructed, which indicates the relation between the size of the dishabituation response and the stimulus distance. For each stimulus distance there is, in addition, a second value of the dishabituation response available (group B), where the change was in the opposite direction, from high to low. The additional values, taken together, again constitute a dishabituation gradient. These two hypothetical gradients are shown in fig. 6.1.

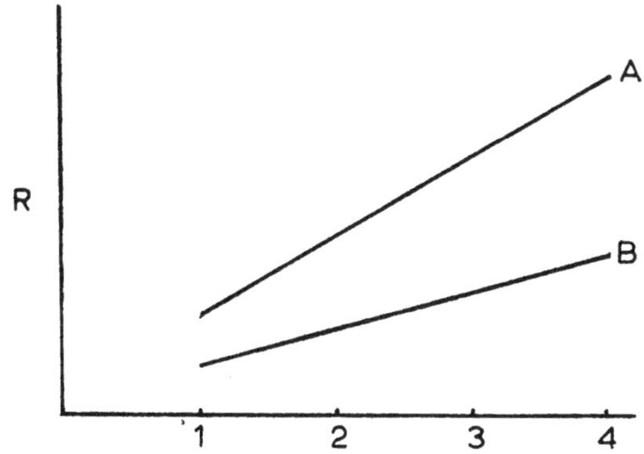

Fig. 6.1. Hypothetical dishabituation gradients

Response size is shown on the Y-axis; stimulus distance on the X-axis. Gradient A is obtained by plotting the stimulus distances from low to high, B from high to low.
According to Sokolov (theory of the neuronal model of the stimulus), the dishabituation response should be a monotonically increasing function of the stimulus distance ('filter curve'). In principle, it makes no difference in which direction the stimulus distances are varied. Put another way, the functions A and B in fig. 6.1 should exhibit the same trend.

The data of tables 6.10 and 6.11 were now subjected to an analysis of variance (in a 2 × 4 design), in which the amplitude of the first response after stimulus change was used as independent variable. If Sokolov's assumptions are correct, the variance due to the factor 'stimulus distance' will be significant, whereas the variance due to the factor 'direction' will not be significant. The results of this analysis are given below.

Source of variance	Sum of squares	df	Mean square	F
Stimulus distance (Sdi)	609.44	3	203.15	< 1.00
Direction (D)	78.02	1	78.02	< 1.00
Sdi × D	905.14	3	301.71	1.26 (n.s.)
Error	15278.30	64	238.72	
Total	16870.89	71		

The results show that the hypothesis stating that the size of the dishabituation response is a monotonically increasing function of the stimulus distance must be rejected. This in fact confirms what visual inspection of the data in tables 6.10 and 6.11 had already made clear; the factor 'direction' produces no significant effect.

Now, it is possible that individual differences in general responsivity have distorted the picture. For this reason a correction for individual differences was made by dividing the particular response size by the first response of the first stimulus sequence (in this first sequence – prior to dishabituation – frequency as such was found to have no significant effect on the response size; see Ch 5.3.4).

The original as well as the corrected values are given in the following table (6.13).

Table 6.13 Original and corrected responses

	Direction: low → high				Direction: high → low			
Sdi	1	2	3	4	1	2	3	4
I	24.1	15.3	13.1	18.1	13.8	23.5	12.0	13.4
II	.756	.695	.510	.720	.497	.720	.627	.317

Sdi = Stimulus distance in octaves
I = original response amplitudes
II = corrected response amplitudes (ratios)

We see that these corrections do not essentially change the picture. Only the effect of the factor 'direction' is somewhat larger ($F = 2.24$; $p < .10$). This is more especially due to the difference in direction for stimulus distance 4 (500 cps ⇆ 8000 cps), the only difference found significant upon application of the test of Kruskal and Wallis for $K = 2$ ($H = 5.7$; $p < .01$).

The same analysis of variance as performed for response amplitude was repeated for response duration and latency.

Response duration

Source of variance	Sum of squares	df	Mean square	F
Stimulus distance (Sdi)	115.89	3	38.63	< 1.00
Direction (D)	72.00	1	72.00	1.78 (n.s.)
Sdi × D	29.44	3	9.82	< 1.00
Error	2588.67	64	40.45	
Total	2806.00	71		

Latency

Source of variance	Sum of squares	df	Mean square	F
Stimulus distance (Sdi)	154.26	3	51.42	5.30 p < .005
Direction (D)	33.35	1	33.35	3.44 p < .10
Sdi × D	172.04	3	57.35	5.91 p < .005
Error	620.67	64	9.70	
Total	980.32	71		

Although we see that the stimulus distance has a significant effect on the response latency, further inspection of tables 6.10 and 6.11 shows that there is no marked systematic relation, mainly as a result of the extreme value of 1.3 in table 6.11 (2000 $\rightleftarrows$ 500 cps).

Habituation rate

The data for the two groups A and B were separately subjected to the non-parametric analysis of variance of Kruskal and Wallis to determine the effect of the stimulus distance on the habituation rate.

Group A: $H = 7.07$ $p < .10$
Group B: $H = .90$ (n.s.)

For each stimulus distance the effect of the factor 'direction' was determined by the Mann-Whitney U-test.

Stimulus distance: 1, $U = 43.0$ (n.s.)
2, $U = 44.5$ (n.s.)
3, $U = 41.5$ (n.s.)
4, $U = 27.0$ $p = .10$

Summary

After initial habituation a change in tone frequency produces dishabituation with regard to both response amplitude and response duration. Shorter latencies were found only in a number of cases.

Sokolov's hypothesis that the degree of dishabituation is a function of the stimulus distance was not confirmed. This latter result is in accord with the findings of Zimny and Schwabe (1965) (See Ch 3.5).

These authors found that after initial habituation to a tone of 500 cps, presentation of a tone of 1000 cps or 4000 cps caused dishabituation. However, no significant differences in the degree of dishabituation were found to occur.

The direction of the stimulus change likewise produces little effect. Neither the distance nor the direction of the stimulus change is found to determine the habituation rate (after dishabituation).

Intersession habituation occurs in respect of all the response properties as well as the habituation rate.

6.4 DISHABITUATION DUE TO CHANGES IN INTENSITY

As in the case of tone frequency, here too the effect of stimulus distance and

Table 6.14 (Group A)

	I	II	III	I	II	III	I	II	III
Stimulus	39 db	39 db	59 db	39 db	39 db	79 db	39 db	39 db	99 db
Amplitude*	30.2	4.3	35.4	22.4	2.3	24.1	23.0	5.6	37.0
Duration	3.0	1.5	2.7	2.9	1.5	3.2	2.7	1.9	3.1
Latency time	1.9	1.9	1.8	1.9	2.3	2.0	1.9	1.9	1.7

* $\triangle$ log C × 1000
I = First response before stimulus change
II = Last ,, ,, ,, ,,
III = First ,, after ,, ,,

Table 6.15 (Group B)

	I	II	III	I	II	III	I	II	III
Stimulus	59 db	59 db	39 db	79 db	79 db	39 db	99 db	99 db	39 db
Amplitude*	32.6	6.0	11.4	63.3	7.8	15.7	93.7	4.1	10.4
Duration	3.1	1.9	2.2	3.7	1'7	2.2	4.6	1.8	1.9
Latency time	1.3	1.5	1.6	1.7	2.0	2.0	1.5	1,8	2.1

* $\triangle$ log C × 1000
I = First response before stimulus change
II = Last ,, ,, ,, ,,
III = First ,, after ,, ,,

the direction of the change was studied. A tone of 2000 cps, duration 0.5 sec, was repeated every 10 sec.

Group A, consisting of 30 subjects, started with an intensity of 39 db. After habituation or 20 stimulations the group was divided into three subgroups, each consisting of 10 subjects. For the first group the intensity was changed to 59 db, for the second to 79 db, and for the third subgroup to 99 db.*

Group B, likewise consisting of 30 subjects, was at once divided into 3 subgroups of 10 subjects each. The first subgroup received an intensity of 59 db, the second of 79 db, and the third subgroup an intensity of 99 db.* After habituation or 20 stimulations the intensity for all the subgroups was changed to 39 db. Apart from the stimulus intensity all the conditions remained the same. The various results are given in tables 6.14, 6.15 and 6.16.

Data

The question as to whether dishabituation occurred was studied by determining both for group A and for group B the number of cases in which the amplitude of the first response after the change in intensity exceeded that of the last response before the change, or alternatively was in excess of zero after complete habituation had occurred. In group A 28 out of 30 subjects showed dishabituation. In group B 26 out of 30 subjects showed dishabituation.

Table 6.16 Habituation rates before (a) and after (b) stimulus change.

	a	b	a	b	a	b
Habituation rate group A	39 db	59 db	39 db	79 db	39 db	99 db
	8.9	6.1	5.8	6.3	7.0	13.0
Habituation rate group B	10.8	5.1	12.1	7.4	18.2	2.4
	59 db	39 db	79 db	39 db	99 db	39 db

Problem specifications and analyses

1. Is the difference between the mean values of the amplitude of the last response before and the first response after dishabituation significant?

* At this intensity the generator showed symptoms of 'leakage', so that the signal in this case cannot be regarded as entirely true.

For each group a separate analysis of variance for repeated measures was performed.

Group A

Source of variance	Sum of squares	df	Mean square	F
Stimulus distance (Sdi)	777.00	2	388.50	1.45 (n.s.)
Ss within Sdi's (Ss)	6452.33	24	268.85	
Dishabituation (D)	11151.41	1	11151.41	36.27 $p < .005$
Sdi × D	345.82	2	172.91	< 1.00
Ss × D	7378.78	24	307.45	
Total	26105.34	53		

Group B

Source of variance	Sum of squares	df	Mean square	F
Stimulus distance (Sdi)	110.38	2	55.19	< 1.00
Ss within Sdi's (Ss)	2983.94	21	142.09	
Dishabituation (D)	623.52	1	623.52	7.26 $p < .025$
Sdi × D	25.79	2	12.90	< 1.00
Ss × D	1803.19	21	85.87	
Total	5546.82	47		

In both groups stimulus change produces a significant increase in amplitude. This effect is most pronounced for group A (weak → strong).

2. Is the difference between the mean values for response duration of the last response before and the first response after dishabituation significant? As with the previous problem, an analysis of variance for repeated measures was performed for both groups.

Group A

Source of variance	Sum of squares*	df	Mean square	F
Stimulus distance (Sdi)	170.23	2	85.12	1.03 (n.s.)
Ss within Sdi's (Ss)	2241.10	27	83.00	
Dishabituation (D)	2801.67	1	2801.67	24.34 $p < .005$
Sdi × D	56.43	2	28.22	< 1.00
Ss × D	3107.90	27	115.11	
Total	8377.33	59		

* Original measures × 10

Group B

Source of variance	Sum of squares	df	Mean square	F
Stimulus distance (Sdi)	1.10	2	0.55	< 1.00
Ss within Sdi's (Ss)	30.45	27	1.33	
Dishabituation (D)	1.98	1	1.98	7.62 $p < .05$
Sdi × D	0.55	2	0.28	1.08 (n.s.)
Ss × D	7.02	27	0.26	
Total	41.10	59		

Stimulus change produces a significant increase in response duration, most markedly in group A.

3. Is the difference between the mean values for response latency of the last response before and the first response after dishabituation significant? Again, an analysis of variance for repeated measures was performed.

Group A

Source of variance	Sum of squares	df	Mean square	F
Stimulus distance (Sdi)	94.90	2	47.45	1.30 (n.s.)
Ss within Sdi's (Ss)	985.45	27	36.50	
Dishabituation (D)	58.02	1	58.02	3.91 $p < .10$
Sdi × D	9.43	2	4.72	< 1.00
Ss × D	401.05	27	14.85	
Total	1548.85	59		

Group B

Source of variance	Sum of squares	df	Mean square	F
Stimulus distance (Sdi)	2.27	2	1.14	3.56 $p < .05$
Ss within Sdi's (Ss)	8.63	27	0.32	
Dishabituation (D)	0.18	1	0.18	4.50 $p < .05$
Sdi × D	0.30	2	0.15	3.75 $p < .05$
Ss × D	1.02	27	0.04	
Total	12.40	59		

Group A exhibits a tendency for the latency to become shorter as a result of stimulus change. On the other hand, group B shows a significant increase in response latency (change-over from strong to weak), an effect which is furthermore significantly influenced by the stimulus distance. Latency increases most with the largest stimulus distance (99 → 39 db).

4. What effect do stimulus distance and direction of change have on the amplitude of the dishabituation response?
In view of the very heterogeneous nature of the variances it was not deemed advisable to perform an analysis of variance, so that a non-parametric test was applied. For a better understanding, the relevant data of tables 6.14 and 6.15 are reproduced below.

Stimulus distance		20 db	40 db	60 db
Direction	weak → strong (A)	35.4	24.1	37.0
	strong → weak (B)	11.4	15.7	10.4

Even cursory inspection shows that the response amplitude is not an increasing function of the stimulus distance. Both for group A and for group B the differences are not significant. Application of the non-parametric analysis of variance of Kruskal and Wallis yielded
for group A: $H = 2.1$ (n.s.)
group B: $H = 1.9$ (n.s.)
For each stimulus distance the differences in direction were likewise subjected to a (two-tailed) test.
Stimulus distance: 20 db $H = 5.9$ $p < .02$ (markedly skew sample distribution)
40 db $t = 1.17$ (n.s.)
60 db $t = 3.45$ $p < .01$
It is to be noted that the value for the 20 db distance of group A (35.4) cannot be considered very representative. The mean responsivity of this subgroup is fairly high. As we have seen, all the subgroups of group A received a tone of 39 db. For the various subgroups the mean size of the first response to this tone was 30.2, 22.4 and 23.0 respectively. Possibly this high value (30.2) has flattered the response amplitude of the first subgroup after stimulus change (59 db), or in other words, the real value for the 20 db distance may be much lower. The possibility therefore exists that for group A (weak to strong) the response size is after all an increasing function of the stimulus distance. Since, however, this argument does not apply to group B (strong to weak), the almost inevitable conclusion is that it is not so much the stimulus distance itself as the absolute intensity which is the operative factor.

In sum, changes in stimulus intensity will cause dishabituation, but the degree of dishabituation is not a function of the stimulus distance. If the change in intensity is in the direction from weak to strong, the absolute intensity of the stimulus will also play a role as OR determinant. This is also in agreement with the findings of Bernstein (1968). In his experiment two groups of subjects received tones of 1000 cps, 60 db and 1000 cps, 90 db respectively. Stimulus duration was 1 sec, and the tones were repeated 15 times. On the 16th trial both groups received a tone of 1000 cps, 75 db. The response amplitude of the + 15 db (60 → 75 db) significantly exceeded that of the — 15 db group (90 → 75 db).
We have before (Ch. 3.5) referred to the work of Kimmel (1960), who found that the OR due to dishabituation upon a change in stimulus intensity was a function of the stimulus distance and the direction of change. Only the latter finding is in accord with what has been said above. In view of the objections that can be raised against Kimmel's experimental methods these findings must be treated with reserve.
It may be noted in passing that on the strength of neurological evidence Thompson (1965) formulated the hypothesis that the generalization from strong to weak tones will be steeper than that from weak to strong stimuli. This would mean that dishabituation in the direction from strong to weak will be greater than in the opposite direction. From the above experimental results, however, the reverse is seen to be the case!

5. What is the effect of the stimulus distance and the direction of the stimulus change on the duration of the dishabituation response?
This question was answered by means of an analysis of variance.

Source of variance	Sum of squares*	df	Mean square	F
Stimulus distance (Sdi)	85.03	2	42.52	< 1.00
Direction (D)	1233.07	1	1233.07	14.06 p < .005
Sdi × D	117.43	2	58.72	< 1.00
Error	4736.40	54	87.71	
Total	6171.93	59		

* Original measures × 10

The difference between the two groups (A and B) in response duration is significant. In group B (strong → weak) the response duration is systematically shorter.

6. What is the effect of the stimulus distance and the direction of the stimulus change on the latency of the dishabituation response?
Again an analysis of variance was performed.

Source of variance	Sum of squares*	df	Mean square	F
Stimulus distance (Sdi)	74.13	2	37.07	2.09 (n.s.)
Direction (D)	1.67	1	1.67	< 1.00
Sdi × D	104.53	2	52.27	2.95 $p < .10$
Error	955.60	54	17.70	
Total	1135.93	59		

* Original measures × 10.

The response latency is apparently not affected by the direction of the stimulus change or by the stimulus distance.

Habituation

7. Does the nature of the dishabituation signal (range and direction of the stimulus distance) affect the habituation rate?
The effect of the stimulus distance was determined by means of the non-parametric analysis of variance of Kruskal and Wallis.
Group A : $H = 14.18$ $p < .01$
Group B : $H = 4.39$ (n.s.)
The significant effect in group A is exclusively due to the value of the 99 db group.
The effect of the factor 'direction' was determined for each stimulus distance by means of the test of Kruskal and Wallis for $k = 2$.

Stimulus distance:	20 db	$H = 0.14$ (n.s.)
	40 db	$H = 0.24$ (n.s.)
	60 db	$H = 14.29$ $p < .01$

Again, the significant difference for the 60 db distance is due to the high value for 99 db in group A.

Intersession habituation

8. Does the response amplitude exhibit intersession habituation?
In group A 30 cases are available which each received 39 db as the first intensity. For the various subgroups the amplitude of the first response showed no significant difference ($H = 0.5$ n.s.).

In group **B** 30 cases were available which each received 39 db as the second intensity (after dishabituation). Again, as had been computed before, there was no significant difference between the subgroups.
The two mean values of the first response, before and after dishabituation, were:
$M_1 = 25.2$ $M_2 = 11.8$ $t = 3.39$ $p < .005$ one-tailed
For the intensity of 59db the mean values were:
$M_1 = 33.6$ $M_2 = 35.4$ No intersession habituation therefore occurs here.
For 79 db $M_1 = 63.3$ $M_2 = 21.7$ ($n = 10$) $t = 2.10$ $p < .05$
For 99 db $M_1 = 93.7$ $M_2 = 37.0$ ($n = 10$) $t = 2.24$ $p < .025$
The occurrence of intersession habituation is thus clearly established. The exception in the case of 59 db is entirely due to the large difference in responsivity between the two groups.

9. Does the response duration exhibit intersession habituation?
To determine this point, an analysis of variance was performed on the data for the 39 db condition.

Source of variance	Sum of squares	df	Mean square	F
Subgroups (S)	93.90	2	46.95	< 1.00
Intersession habituation (I)	897.07	1	897.07	8.51 $p < .01$
S × I	14.43	2	7.22	< 1.00
Error	5689.20	54	105.36	
Total	6694.60	59		

For 59 db $M_1 = 3.1$ $M_2 = 2.7$ ($n = 10$) $t = 0.11$ (n.s.)
For 79 db $M_1 = 3.7$ $M_2 = 3.2$,, $t = 0.11$ (n.s.)
For 99 db $M_1 = 4.6$ $M_2 = 3.1$,, $t = 0.49$ (n.s.)

In general, intersession habituation (a decrease in response duration) occurs. However, this tendency assumes significance only for the 39 db group (under this condition 30 observations were available).

10. Does the response latency exhibit intersession habituation?
Again, an analysis of variance was performed on the data of the 39 db condition.

Source of variance	Sum of squares	df	Mean square	F
Subgroups (S)	132.23	2	66.12	4.09 $p < .05$.
Intersession habituation (I)	17.07	1	17.07	1.06 (n.s.)
$S \times I$	59.43	2	29.72	1.84 (n.s.)
Error	872.60	54	16.16	
Total	1081.33	59		

For 59 db $M_1 = 1.3$ $M_2 = 1.8$ $t = -0.32$ (n.s.)
For 79 db $M_1 = 1.7$ $M_2 = 2.0$ $t = -0.19$ (n.s.)
For 99 db $M_1 = 1.5$ $M_2 = 1.7$ $t = -0.12$ (n.s.)

Although the general tendency is towards longer latencies, the effect nowhere becomes significant.

11. Does the habituation rate exhibit intersession habituation?
For each of the four intensities the difference in habituation rate was subjected to the Wilcoxon test.

39 db $M_1 = 7.2$ $M_2 = 5.0$ $z = 1.64$ $p = .05$
59 db $M_1 = 10.8$ $M_2 = 5.4$ $T = 12$ $p < .10$
79 db $M_1 = 12.1$ $M_2 = 6.3$ $T = 13$ $p < .10$
99 db $M_1 = 18.6$ $M_2 = 13.0$ $T = 1$ $p < .005$

The habituation rate decreases as a result of intersession habituation. After stimulus modification habituation is attained more quickly than before the change-over.

12. Is the change in pre-stimulus level due to stimulus modification significant?
To this end, the pre-stimulus levels of the last response before and the second response after stimulus change were compared.
For group A these values were .738 and .771 respectively. This difference was significant ($F = 64.64, p < .005$). The stimulus distance produced no significant effect. For group B the mean values were .917 and .915. The difference was not significant ($F < 1.00$).

Summary

Changes in stimulus intensity, whether from weak to strong or from strong to weak, produce dishabituation, which manifests itself in a (significant) increase in the amplitude and duration of the response. This process is not affected by the degree of change (stimulus distance). As regards the response latency, this is found to decrease significantly in the direction from weak to strong but to increase significantly if the change-over is from strong to weak. In the latter case the effect is influenced by the degree of change (stimulus distance). This Lt increase is at variance with the usual effect upon dishabituation, which is one of Lt shortening. In this case the effect of the absolute stimulus intensity is apparently predominant.

A comparison of the dishabituation responses shows that their amplitude is not a function of the stimulus distance if the change-over is from strong to weak. If, on the other hand, the change is from weak to strong, the response size probably *is* an increasing function of the stimulus distance. In view also of the fact that in the change-over from strong to weak the responses for each of the stimulus distances are smaller than when the change is in the opposite direction, the obvious conclusion seems to be that the size of the dishabituation response upon intensity modification is not a function of the stimulus distance. If under the condition weak → strong such a relation should occur, this is merely due to the fact that the size of the OR is a function of the absolute intensity.

These results are at variance with the views of Sokolov (1960) and Thompson (1965), which in fact are mutually exclusive, but in agreement with the findings of Bernstein (1968) and probably those of Kimmel (1960).

The data on response duration point in the same direction, that is, while showing no relation with the stimulus distance, they do exhibit the effect of the direction of change. The response latency is found to be affected by neither of these factors.

Intersession habituation was determined by establishing for each separate intensity the difference between the first response before and the first response after stimulus change. As far as response amplitude is concerned, the effect was found to occur at all the intensities apart from the 59 db group. As regards response duration, intersession habituation could be demonstrated only at the 39 db intensity. The response latency was not subject to this effect. In the case of the 39 db as well as the 99 db stimulus, the habituation process was found to proceed more quickly.

Finally, it was found that only if the change-over is from weak to strong does the pre-stimulus level (log C) increase significantly. This provides further evidence for the view advanced by us that in this case the absolute stimulus intensity determines the response.

7 AN EXPERIMENTAL INVESTIGATION OF OTHER OR PROPERTIES

7.1 PERCEPTUAL EXPECTATION AS AN OR DETERMINANT

Whenever a stimulus sequence containing two different kinds of stimuli is presented, the subject will generally discern a certain structure in the sequence. This also applies to a randomized sequence, since in any finite series there is always a limit to the number of successive occurrences of the same stimulus. To the observer this limit may appear to constitute something like the principle of the sequence. Put another way, if a subject believes that a particular stimulus cannot occur more than three times in a row, he will expect the other stimulus on the next trial. If then the original stimulus is presented on that trial, the subject will experience an incongruity between the actual and the expected stimulus, and this incongruity elicits an OR.

With a view to testing this assumption, various sequences of increasing complexity were composed on the following principle. Each sequence was characterized by a particular maximum of the number of successive trials on which one of the two stimuli could occur. In the four sequences used this maximum was 1, 2, 3 or 4, and any sequence with a given maximum also contained all the values below that maximum.

The sequences were composed of two tones, T_1 (1000 cps, 60 db) and T_2 (4000 cps, 54 db). Each sequence consisted of a total of 40 tones, both tones occurring with roughly the same frequency. The duration of the tones, which were presented every 10 sec, was 0.5 sec.

In the first sequence (S_q1) the two tones were simply alternated (T_1, T_2, T_1, T_2 etc).

In the second sequence (S_q2) successive occurrences of T_1 were limited to two. This pattern (... T_2, T_1, T_1, T_2 ...) occurred seven times in all, while the other seven presentations of T_1 regularly alternated with the T_2 (... T_2, T_1, T_2 ...).

In the third sequence (S_q3) the maximum of successive occurrences of T_1

was three. The characteristic patterns in this sequence were: three times the combination . . . T_2, T_1, T_2. . . , four times the combination. . . T_2, T_1, T_1, T_2 . . . and three times the combination . . . T_2, T_1, T_1, T_1, T_2 . . . .

In the fourth and last sequence (S_q4) the patterns were: three times . . . T_2, T_1, T_2 . . ., twice . . . T_2, T_1, T_1, T_2 . . ., once . . . T_2, T_1, T_1, T_1, T_2 . . . and three times. . . T_2, T_1, T_1, T_1, T_1, T_2 . . . .

Each sequence began with T_1 and ended with T_2, except S_q3, where owing to faulty registration on the tape used for operating the tone generator, trial 39 contained the last T_2. Each sequence was presented to 10, always different, subjects. Completion of the sequence was immediately followed by 10 presentations of T_1 (trials 41–50).

To make the subjects concentrate on the configuration of the sequence, T_2 was signalized by pairing it with a motor reaction. To this end, subjects were instructed to press a key on hearing T_2. We shall revert to this signalization in the appropriate place. On being questioned, subjects afterwards reported that their attention had nevertheless been insufficiently concentrated, or rather had been concentrated on less relevant aspects, notably the temporal ones.

Now it was assumed that subjects would develop a measure of insight into the structure of the sequence. Once this insight is present, there will be a certain moment, depending on the nature of the preceding sequence, when during the second phase of only T_1 presentations (trials 41–50) the subject experiences an incongruity, with a resulting OR. This effect will be studied separately for each of the sequences.

Sq1 The last trial (40) consisted of a T_2. The next T_2 will therefore be expected on trial 42, so that it may be assumed that the response to trial 42 will exceed that to trial 41. Possibly the incongruity effect will in some degree extend to trial 43.

The table (7.1) below shows the mean response amplitude ($\triangle \log C \times 1000$).

Table 7.1

Trial	39	40	41	42	43
Response	2.0	2.5	5.2	16.3	8.6

The difference between trials 41 and 42 was subjected to the t-test for related samples and found to show low significance ($t = 1.51$; $p < .10$). It is to be noted, however, that the mean response amplitude to trial 41 is greatly distorted by one extreme measure, as can be seen from a comparison with the mean value for trial 39. This lower value of 2.0 is a much better estimate, since the mean value for trials 33, 35, 37 and 39 is 2.1. A test of the difference between trial 39 and 42 yields $t = 2.58$ $p < .025$. Questioning revealed that 6 of the 10 subjects had perceived the structure of the sequence, but the findings on this score are not entirely in line with the observed responses.

Sq2 In this sequence, with maximally two successive occurrences of T_1, the incongruity effect is to be expected on trial 43, possibly extending to trial 44. The table (7.2) shows the mean response amplitudes.

Table 7.2

Trial	40	41	42	43	44
Response	4.4	2.1	2.0	2.0	2.2

On trial 43 only one response was given which clearly exceeded the previous one (from 0 to 15). No difference is therefore observed between trials 42 and 43, and possibly 44.
Nevertheless 4 of the 10 subjects were found to show some understanding of the sequence structure.

Sq3 In this sequence the incongruity effect may be expected on trial 43, and possibly 44. The observations are given below.

Table 7.3

Trial	39	40	41	42	43	44
Response	7.8	6.3	3.4	0.8	3.6	2.5

The difference between trials 42 and 43 is significant ($t = 2.56$ $p < .025$) and so is the difference between trials 42 and 44 ($t = 2.18$ $p < .05$). In view of the preceding trials, however, it is questionable whether these are real differences. If one takes the average of trial, 40, 41 and 42, the effect disappears completely. Two of the ten subjects were found to have perceived the principle of this sequence.

Sq4 An incongruity effect may be expected on trial 45, and possibly 46. The observations are given below.

Table 7.4

Trial	40	41	42	43	44	45	46
Response	10.0	5.4	6.8	2.6	1.5	2.6	2.5

The differences between trials 44 and 45, and between 44 and 46, were not significant. Two of the ten subjects showed some insight into the structure of the sequence.

If we now correlate for all the sequences the perception or non-perception of the sequence structure with the occurrence or non-occurrence of a (larger) response, we get the following picture.

	Response —	*Response* +
Principle +	7	7
Perceived —	16	10

As we see, the two variables show little correlation. There are a number of cases where insight into the sequence is clearly accompanied by an OR occurrence. Most subjects, however, hardly realized what was going on. We find therefore that no general confirmation has been obtained for the hypotheses formulated by us. Only for the simplest sequence is the effect found to be significant.

7.2 THE SIGNALIZATION PHENOMENON

Signalization is the acquisition of signal value; as a rule, this process is set in train by a verbal instruction. The OR's to signal stimuli are held to exceed those to non-signal stimuli and to habituate less quickly.

When in a given experimental situation a conditioned response (CR) becomes established, reciprocal inhibition (Ch 2.2.3) occurs. That is to say, the initially large OR's to the signal stimulus will, for the purpose of stimulus evaluation, to some extent inhibit the CR. This is said to be more especially the case with so-called 'voluntary motor conditioning' (VMC).

As signalization advances, the OR becomes smaller and its inhibitory effect decreases, with resulting facilitation of the voluntary motor response (VMR). In the simple case of a non-complex reaction task (a-reaction), the RT shortening that occurs in the course of the experiment, and which is regarded as a training effect, could therefore be the result of a decrease in reciprocal inhibition.

To determine whether and to what extent these phenomena occur, we conducted some experiments which will be discussed in the following section.

7.2.1 Signalization in a simple RT task

In a simple RT experiment 120 subjects were required to react as quickly as possible to a tone of 500 cps, 56db. (The data are derived from an experiment to be discussed in the next section.) The tone, repeated every 20 sec, was terminated by the subject's reaction. Simultaneously the GSR was measured. The entire series consisted of 25 trials. On the 25th trial 117 of the 120 subjects were still found to respond to the tone with a distinct OR. The habituation rate therefore was at least 25.

Although no adequate control group was available, some degree of comparison is possible with data from another experiment conducted by us (see Ch 6.3). There the mean habituation rate of 40 subjects to a tone of 500 cps, 56 db, duration 0.5 sec, and repeated every 10 sec, was found to be 10.1. While admittedly the interval was shorter in this case, we have seen in Ch 5.3.2 that the longer interval produces only a slight increase in habituation rate. These data already go to show that stimuli with signal value much longer continue to evoke an OR.

Table 7.5 presents values of the variables RT, $\triangle$ log C, and the pre-stimulus level log C for the 2nd and the 25th trials (mean values for 117 subjects, since three subjects had a habituation rate < 25).

Table 7.5 The course of the signalizing process

Trial	2	6	25
RT	0.29	0.26	0.28
$\triangle$ log C	25		14
log C	0.995		1.001

For RT the value of the 6th trial has also been included, since inspection of the data showed that on the 6th trial the RT attained its minimum value. The values of $\triangle$ log C have been multiplied by 10^3.
The decrease in $\triangle$ log C was found to be significant ($t = 7.63$; $p < .001$); the change in log C was not significant ($t = 1.28$; $p > .10$).

To determine whether the RT exhibited a significant trials effect, an analysis of variance for repeated measures was performed.

Source of variance	Sum of squares	df	Mean square	F
Trials (T)	541.70	2	270.85	8.85 $p < .005$
Subjects (Ss)	9069.32	116	78.18	2.55 $p < .005$
T × Ss	7100.97	232	30.61	
Total	16711.99	350		

Since the multiple range test of Duncan can only be applied to independent observations, the data were randomized. This was done by selecting the 2nd trial of the first subject, the 6th trial of the second subject, the 25th trial of the third subject, after which again the 2nd trial of the fourth subject was selected, etc. The observations thus obtained were subjected to the test of Duncan. The difference between the 2nd and the 6th as well as between the 2nd and the 25th trial proved to be significant ($p < .05$); the difference between the 6th and the 25th trial was not significant.

With due reserve it may therefore be concluded that there is a certain reciprocal relation; in the course of the process the OR to the signal stimulus becomes smaller, while the efficiency of the motor behavior increases somewhat.

7.2.2 Differential signalization

In the previous experiment the effect of signalization upon repetition of the same stimulus was studied. The question may be asked how signalization proceeds in sequences consisting of a number of stimuli, to only one of which the subject is required to react ('differential signalization'). One part of the stimuli acquires signal value, the other part does not.

It may be assumed, therefore, that the OR's to the signal stimuli will be larger and will habituate less quickly than the OR's to the non-signal stimuli. A sequence like this, consisting of two kinds of stimuli, may show greater or less regularity in the alternation of the stimuli. Less regularity means more uncertainty as regards the occurrence of the signal stimulus. Uncertainty is an OR determinant. It follows that as the irregularity in a sequence increases, the habituation of the OR's to the signal stimuli will proceed more slowly.

These hypotheses were tested on the data collected in the experiments on perceptual expectation. For a description of the stimulus materials we therefore refer to Ch 7.1. There were four sequences, Sq1, Sq2, Sq3 and Sq4, showing increasing irregularity. T_2 was the signal stimulus, T_1 the non-signal stimulus. The GSR was measured on all the trials; RT was not determined.

For each sequence the mean values of the GSR to signal and non-signal stimuli were calculated and the difference between the two tested. The table below (7.6) shows the obtained values ($\triangle$ log C $\times$ 1000).

Table 7.6 Mean OR's to signal and non-signal stimuli

Sequence	Signal stimuli	Non-signal stimuli	t	p
Sq1	65.9	49.8	1.81	<.05
Sq2	88.1	52.7	3.25	<.005
Sq3	112.6	84.2	2.34	<.025
Sq4	99.2	67.8	4.23	<.005

The difference between signal and non-signal stimuli is thus found to be significant for all the sequences.

The second hypothesis, to the effect that the responses to signal stimuli decrease less quickly with increasing irregularity of the sequence, was tested by means of a simple analysis of variance. The sequence effect was found to be significant ($F = 5.72$; $p < .01$). The differences between the non-signal stimuli are not significant ($F < 1.00$).

Although the difference between the signal stimuli of the four sequences is significant, the value of Sq4 is not in line with the hypothesis. This value ought to exceed that of Sq3. This discrepancy must probably be attributed to differences in physiological responsivity between the groups. This appears quite clearly from the size of the first responses of the various sequences. (All the sequences started with a non-signal stimulus.) These mean values for Sq1 through Sq4 were: 33.2, 29.7, 35.1 and 23.7. When a correction for this difference is made in the response to the signal stimuli by dividing these responses by the size of the first response of the particular sequence, the following values are obtained:

.320 .481 .531 .597

The corrected responses completely bear out the assumption that the size of the OR to signal stimuli is an increasing function of the irregularity in the sequence. For completeness' sake we finally determined whether there were systematic differences in the mean pre-stimulus levels (log C). As appears from the table (7.7) below, this was not the case.

Table 7.7 Mean pre-stimulus levels

	Sq1	Sq2	Sq3	Sq4
Non-signal stimuli	11.30	10.23	10.75	11.21
Signal stimuli	11.31	10.23	10.78	11.21

7.3 THE INHIBITORY FUNCTION OF THE OR

In Ch 2.1 the inhibitory function of the OR has already been defined. The occurrence of an OR inhibits the 'ongoing behavior'. It seems natural to assume that the degree of inhibition will be a function of the size of the OR. This hypothesis was tested in the following experiment.

In a simple RT experiment 120 subjects were instructed to react as quickly as possible to a tone (500 cps, 56 db with a 20 sec interval). After 25 trials (the data of this first phase were analyzed in the previous section) the subjects were divided into five subgroups. For the first subgroup the experimental condition was without interruption continued with five extra trials. On trials 26 through 30 the other subgroups received – without previous announcement – a tone of 1000 cps (60 db), 2000 cps (59 db), 4000 cps (54 db) or 8000 cps (65 db).

For the various subgroups the mean RT's were determined of trials 24 and 25, as well as of trials 26 and 27. These values are shown in the table below (7.8).

Table 7.8 Reaction times before and after dishabituation

	Subgroups				
	500 cps	1000 cps	2000 cps	4000 cps	8000 cps
Mean RT (trials 24 and 25)	0.30	0.27	0.28	0.29	0.26
Mean RT (trials 26 and 27)	0.31	0.31	0.34	0.35	0.31

For each subgroup the difference between the two mean values was tested for significance:

500 cps	$t = .85$	$p > .20$
1000 cps	$t = 1.73$	$p < .05$
2000 cps	$t = 1.42$	$p < .10$
4000 cps	$t = 2.79$	$p < .005$
8000 cps	$t = 2.62$	$p < .01$

On the strength of these data it may be concluded that stimulus change produces a certain degree of inhibition, which manifests itself in RT prolongation. To determine whether the degree of inhibition was a function of the degree of stimulus dissimilarity an analysis of variance was applied to the differences between the RT's before and after stimulus change. The effect of the degree of stimulus dissimilarity proved not significant ($F < 1.00$).

This is not to say that the degree of inhibition is not a function of the size of the OR. To determine this point, the GSR data must be further analyzed.

The table below (7.9) shows the mean GSR's ($\times$ 1000) for the 25th and 26th trials.

Table 7.9 GSR's *before and after dishabituation*

	Subgroups				
	500	1000	2000	4000	8000
Mean GSR trial 25	12.5	13.5	12.2	12.5	16.2
Mean GSR trial 26	9.3	33.0	20.6	25.4	37.4

The differences between the two mean values were tested for each subgroup.

500 cps	$t = -1.54$	$p < .10$
1000 cps	$t = 5.43$	$p < .005$
2000 cps	$t = 3.78$	$p < .005$
4000 cps	$t = 5.96$	$p < .005$
8000 cps	$t = 3.53$	$p < .005$

The 500 cps group clearly shows the effect of continued dishabituation. The differences for the other groups are highly significant; in each subgroup the stimulus change has therefore produced an OR.

However, the degree of dishabituation is not found to be an increasing function of the stimulus dissimilarity, as posited by Sokolov's filter model.* This may provide the explanation for the fact that the RT increase is likewise not an increasing function of the stimulus difference.

The only conclusion that can be drawn from the foregoing is that stimulus change during an RT task evokes an OR which is accompanied by a certain degree of inhibition of the motor behavior.

7.4 Summary

The results of this chapter may be summed up as follows. Manipulation of the factor 'perceptual expectation' was found to be less simple than had originally been supposed. Only in the case of the most elementary sequence (Sq 1) could the subjects be said to show real insight, which was mostly accompanied by OR occurrences. The problem primarily hinges on how to instil a certain perceptual expectation. Only with the first sequence was instilment of a pattern of perceptual expectation achieved. In this case the hypothesis that an OR will occur could be confirmed. For the more complex sequences it was not found possible to instil a perceptual expectation pattern.

For all cases signalization could be demonstrated in the form of larger OR's and delayed habituation. An important point in this respect was that in differential signalization the degree of signalizing (the size of the OR and delay of habituation) was found to be a positive function of the irregularity or uncertainty in the sequence. It was further demonstrated that a somewhat increased efficiency in the performance of an RT task was accompanied by a decrease of the OR to the signal stimulus.

Finally, it was found that stimulus change in an RT task evoked an OR, which was accompanied by a certain degree of inhibition of the motor behavior. Here neither the size of the OR nor the degree of inhibition, measured as RT prolongation, was a function of the distance between the original and the modified stimulus.

These latter findings are not in agreement with what was to be expected on the basis of Sokolov's filter model.

* Sokolov's filter model is primarily concerned with non-signal stimuli. Since in our case signal stimuli are involved, it could perhaps be supposed that the filter model does not apply to signal stimuli. Actually, however, the filter model was found not to be applicable either when non-signal stimuli were used (see Ch 6).

8 HABITUATION AND DISHABITUATION TO COMPLEX STIMULI

In Ch 4.1.1b the stimuli used for this purpose have been described in general terms. These stimuli are of a more complex structure than the purely sensory stimuli used thus far. In our case they are sequences of numbers and words. The central issue is whether after repeated presentations of stimuli ordered along a certain dimension OR habituation will occur and, conversely, whether stimuli that are clearly outside this dimension will cause dishabituation. To permit a more detailed exploration of this problem we conducted the following experiments.

8.1 NUMBER SEQUENCES

The number sequences used were composed according to certain underlying principles. Now the assumption was that during the successive presentations of the terms of the sequence OR habituation would occur in accordance with the principles of the sequence, or to put it another way, that the invariant property of the stimulation, the principle of the sequence, would become fixed in the neuronal model of the stimulation.

If now the principle or the regularity of the sequence is at a certain moment disrupted by an extraneous term, *i.e.* by stimulus change, dishabituation will result. A total of four sequences was composed which showed an increasing degree of complexity. Each sequence of numbers was presented to 10 subjects by auditory means (one number every 10 sec). Naturally, successive presentations make it more difficult for the subject to discover the principle than when the numbers are presented simultaneously. Measured were response amplitude ($\triangle \log C \times 1000$) and duration. Significance was tested throughout by the Wilcoxon test.

8.1.1 The first sequence

This sequence consisted of all even numbers from 2 through 34 in their natural order. The stimulus change consisted in the number 27 being inserted between 26 and 28.

Data

Table 8.1 First sequence

	Response	
	Amplitude	Duration
I	30.5	2.9
II	3.5	1.6
III	8.5	2.0
IV	4.0	1.5

I = First response
II = Mean value of the last three responses
III = First response after stimulus change
IV = Second response after stimulus change, *i.e.* upon continuation of the original sequence

There is evident habituation; the difference between I and II is significant. All the subjects gave a dishabituation response.

Decrease in amplitude: $T = 0$ $p < .005$
Decrease in response duration: $T = 1$ $p < .005$.
The effect of the stimulus change (difference between II and III) was significant for the amplitude, $T = 7.5$ $p < .025$, but not significant for the response duration, $T = 18.5$ $p = .18$.

All the subjects had perceived the stimulus change. Upon continuation of the original sequence (IV) the effect of the stimulus change no longer plays a part.

8.1.2 The second sequence

This sequence was formed by the multiplication table of three (3, 6, 9, etc) continued through 48. The stimulus change consisted in the number 47 being inserted between the terms 45 and 48.

Data

Table 8.2 Second sequence

	Response	
	Amplitude	Duration
I	22.3	2.6
II	1.5	1.2
III	12.8	2.2
IV	4.2	1.4

I = First response
II = Mean value of the last three responses
III = First response after stimulus change
IV = Second response after stimulus change, *i.e.* upon continuation of the original sequence

There is a significant habituation effect. For the decrease in both amplitude and response duration we find $T = 0\ p < .005$. The stimulus change clearly causes dishabituation in all the subjects. For the increase in amplitude we find $T = 0\ p < .005$, for the increase in response duration $T = 3\ p < .025$. The dishabituation effect is found to persist upon continuation of the original sequence, the difference between II and IV being significant, $T = 1\ p < .01$.

The stimulus change was perceived by all the subjects.

8.1.3 The third sequence

This sequence, which started with one, was composed of terms obtained by continually adding three to the previous term, which gave 1, 4, 7, 10, etc,

Data

Table 8.3 Third sequence

	Response	
	Amplitude	Duration
I	26.7	2.7
II	1.2	0.9
III	9.4	1.2
IV	5.5	1.4

I = First response
II = Mean value of the last three responses
III = First response after stimulus change
IV = Second response after stimulus change, *i.e.* upon continuation of the original sequence

through 46. The stimulus change was realized by inserting the number 45 between the terms 43 and 46.
The habituation effect is significant. For the amplitude we find $T = 0$ $p < .005$, for the response duration $T = 0$ $p < .01$.

Five of the ten subjects gave a distinct dishabituation response. For the total group, however, the difference between II and III was not significant. The effect of the stimulus change apparently persists upon continuation of the original sequence since the difference in response duration between II and IV attains a certain significance ($T = 6.5$ $p = .05$).

Despite the results, nine out of ten subjects were found to have perceived the stimulus change.

8.1.4 The fourth sequence

This sequence, the most complex of the four, likewise started with the number one. The difference between two successive terms started at one and continually increased by one, producing the sequence: 1, 2, 4, 7, 11, 16, etc through 121. The stimulus change was realized by inserting the number 116 between the terms 106 and 121.

Data

Table 8.4 Fourth sequence

	Response	
	Amplitude	Duration
I	29.8	2.8
II	1.8	1.3
III	2.3	0.6
IV	0.3	0.6

I = First response
II = Mean value of the last three responses
III = First response after stimulus change
IV = Second response after stimulus change, *i.e.* upon continuation of the original sequence

As in the case of the preceding sequences, the habituation effect is significant. For the decrease in amplitude we find $T = 0$ $p < .005$, for the decrease in response duration $T = 1.5$ $p < .025$.

The stimulus change causes no significant increase in amplitude or response duration. Only two subjects made a dishabituation response.

The stimulus change was perceived by six of the ten subjects, including one of the two dishabituation cases.

Summary

In all four different sequences stimulus repetition produced a significant habituation effect. In the first two sequences a significant dishabituation effect could be observed after stimulus change. In both cases the stimulus change was perceived by all the subjects.

While the number of subjects who perceived the stimulus change was smaller in the last two sequences, the decrease was not so pronounced as the smaller dishabituation effects would seem to suggest. In the third sequence *five* subjects exhibited dishabituation, but *nine* (including these five) perceived the stimulus change. In the fourth sequence only two subjects made a dishabituation response, while the stimulus change was perceived by five subjects, including one who exhibited dishabituation.

It is clear that these two entities, dishabituation and perception of the stimulus change, do not exhibit a simple, direct correlation. The data seem to indicate that while perception of the stimulus change is a condition for dishabituation, it is not in fact the only condition. There is one exception to this rule: in the fourth sequence one case of dishabituation occurs where the subject does not report having perceived the stimulus change. No undue importance should be attached to this finding.

A parallel is afforded by the once debated issue as to whether autonomic conditioning was accompanied by awareness of the stimulus relations. The original view that no insight or awareness was needed was later shown to have been based on a not entirely adequate method of experimentation.

Chatterjee and Eriksen (1960, 1962) and Shean (1968) have demonstrated that introspection does not produce altogether reliable evidence. The experiments of these authors show that, if the instruction is manipulated as variable, the insight into the stimulus relations shows a positive correlation with the outcome of the conditioning process. These results also proved to be in accord with the findings on the questionnaire administered on conclusion of the experiment. A negative introspection finding, as obtained in our case, therefore does not necessarily indicate absence of insight into the stimulus relation.

8.2 WORD SEQUENCES

In general, people react primarily to the meaning rather than to the sound of words. With a view to further exploration of various aspects of this phenomenon, a number of (Dutch) word sequences were composed. By means of these the question was studied whether and in what manner habituation and dishabituation manifest themselves in this case. The four types of sequences used exhibited different stimulus invariances of the following nature:

1. Identical vowel sounds
2. Repetition of the same stimulus word
3. Words with particular semantic scale values
4. Identical semantic relations within pairs of words.

Each group or subgroup again consisted of ten subjects.

8.2.1

To determine the effect of identical (vowel) sounds two different sequences were used.

a) The first sequence consisted of Dutch words composed of two sounds, the latter always being a long a, phonetically [a.], such as 'pa', 'ra', 'la', etc, 10 words in all. The stimulus change on the 11th and 12th trials consisted of a vowel change, from a [a.] to o [o.] as in 'po', 'ro', 'lo'. In view of the marked predominance of the [a.] sound in these words (invariant characteristic of the stimulations), it was postulated that habituation would largely be in respect of the vowel sound, which should produce distinct dishabituation on presentation of the stimulus change. Again response amplitude and duration were measured (table 8.5).

Table 8.5

	Amplitude*	Duration
I	23.6	2.1
II	2.9	1.1
III	5.9	1.2
IV	6.7	1.2

* $\triangle \log C \times 1000$
I = First response
II = Mean value of the last three responses
III = First response after stimulus change
IV = Second response after stimulus change

Significance was again determined by the Wilcoxon test.
In both respects, amplitude and duration, the habituation effect is significant. For amplitude: $T = 0$ $p < .005$; for response duration: $T = 1$ $p < .025$.
The difference between II and III, dishabituation, is not significant ($p > .10$), whereas there *is* a significant difference between II and IV, at least in amplitude ($T = 1$ $p < .025$).
All the subjects were found to have perceived the stimulus change, *i.e.* the transition from [a.] to [o.], but many were very vague as to the precise moment of its occurrence. We got a strong impression that some subjects had only perceived the change on its second presentation, which could account for the significance of the dishabituation effect on the 12th trial.

b) The second sequence could in a sense be regarded as a variant of the last one. The words consisted of three sounds making up one syllable, the second sound always being short a (pronounced roughly as in English 'but'). The subjects received 20 such words as 'pap', 'nat', 'mak', 'vat', after which on the 21st trial 'pop' was presented. The sound change was therefore not quite so pronounced as in the preceding sequence. The response data are given below. (table 8.6)

Table 8.6

	Amplitude*	Duration
I	31.5	2.9
II	1.9	0.4
III	1.5	0.5

* $\Delta \log C \times 1000$
I = First response
II = Mean value of the last three responses
III = Response after stimulus change

The habituation effect is significant; both for amplitude and duration we find $T = 0$ $p < .005$. A dishabituation response was given in only one of the ten cases. All the same, seven subjects, including the cases of dishabituation, were afterwards able to reproduce the stimulus change. Apparently the difference in stimulation is too small to cause distinct dishabituation.

8.2.2

The next problem studied was the way in which after repeated presentations of a given stimulus word (habituation) dishabituation developed upon presentation of a synonym and an antonym. To control for sequence effects, one group of subjects received first the synonym and then the antonym, while the reverse order was used for the other group. If reaction is primarily to the meaning of the stimulus words, presentation of an antonym may be expected to cause more dishabituation than a synonym.

In a sense, this line of reasoning links on directly to the statement of Luria and Vinogradova (1959) that a signalized OR will be generalized to stimuli related in meaning to the original stimulus. In the present case, therefore, the issue is one of generalization of habituation, and an attempt will be made to differentiate between various semantic relationships. The three different sequences used will be discussed below under a, b and c.

a) The first sequence consisted of 16 presentations of the (Dutch) word 'kat' (Eng. cat), after which the new stimuli 'hond' (dog) and 'poes' (puss) were presented in either order. The response data are given in table 8.7.

Table 8.7

	Amplitude				Response duration			
	I	II	III	IV	I	II	III	IV
A	34.2	2.0	9.4	8.0	3.2	1.1	1.8	1.5
B	21.1	2.6	7.6	11.0	2.5	1.2	1.8	2.0
C	27.6	2.3	8.6	9.5	2.9	1.2	1.8	1.8

I = First response to 'kat'
II = Mean value of the last three responses to 'kat'
III = Responses to 'hond'
IV = Response to 'poes'

A = Order 'hond', 'poes'
B = Order 'poes', 'hond'
C = Mean value of A and B

The habituation effects are significant.

Group A: Amplitude $T = 0, p < .005$
Response duration $T = 0, p < .005$

Group B: Amplitude $T = 0, p < .005$
Response duration $T = 0, p < .005$

Also, there is evident dishabituation due to stimulus change. The increase in amplitude is significant for both stimulus words ('hond' and 'poes') in either order of presentation.

Amplitude

Group A:	change-over II → III	:	$T = 0$	$p < .005$
	change-over II → IV	:	$T = 1.5$	$p < .025$
Group B:	change-over II → III	:	$T = 0$	$p < .005$
	change-over II → IV	:	$T = 0$	$p < .005$

Response duration

Group A:	change-over II → III	:	$T = 11.5$	n.s.
	change-over II → IV	:	$T = 0$	$p = .025$
Group B:	change-over II → III	:	$T = 3.5$	$p < .025$
	change-over II → IV	:	$T = 3$	$p < .025$

The results under C show that the respective degrees of dishabituation caused by the two new stimulus words 'hond' and 'poes' are not affected by their different semantic values. The difference in amplitude is not significant ($T = 48$).
If subjects' reaction had been primarily to the meaning of the word 'kat', presentation of 'hond' could have been expected to cause more dishabituation than 'poes', which clearly is not the case. On the other hand, no generalization of habituation to the word 'poes' occurs. Only the stimulus change *per se* apparently determines the reaction of these groups. Of the 20 subjects 18, including all cases of dishabituation, were able to reproduce the stimulus change exactly.

b) The second sequence consisted of sixteen presentations of the Dutch word 'donker' (Eng. dark) after which the new stimulus words 'licht' (light) and 'duister' (murky) were presented in either order, The response data are given in table 8.8.

The habituation effects are significant.

Group A:	Amplitude	$T = 0$,	$p < .005$
	Response duration	$T = 0$,	$p < .005$
Group B:	Amplitude	$T = 0$,	$p < .005$
	Response duration	$T = 0$,	$p < .005$

The first response after stimulus change clearly exhibits dishabituation.

Table 8.8

	Amplitude				Response duration			
	I	II	III	IV	I	I	III	IV
A	53.5	1.6	13.4	9.8	3.0	0.8	2.0	1.8
B	28.9	2.8	3.8	16.3	3.1	0.9	1.3	2.3
C	41.2	2.2	8.6	13.1	3.1	0.9	1.7	2.1

I = First response to 'donker'
II = Mean value of the last three responses to 'donker'
III = Response to 'licht'
IV = Response to 'duister'

A = Order 'licht', 'duister'
B = Order 'duister', 'licht'
C = Mean value of A and B

Amplitude

Group A: change-over II → III : $T = 0$ $p < .005$
change-over II → IV : $T = 9$ $p < .03$
Group B: change-over II → III : $T = 13.5$ n.s.
change-over II → IV : $T = 0$ $p < .005$

Response duration

Group A: change-over II → III : $T = 3.5$ $p < .10$
change-over II → IV : $T = 0$ $p < .025$
Group B: change-over II → III : $T = 10$ n.s.
change-over II → IV : $T = 2$ $p < .10$

Again the supposition that the word of opposite meaning would cause the most dishabituation is not fulfilled. The difference between III and IV under C is not significant ($T = 72$). All twenty subjects correctly reported the stimulus change.

c) The third sequence consisted of sixteen presentations of the word 'traag' (Eng. sluggish), after which the words 'snel' (fast) and 'langzaam' (slow) were given. The response data are presented in table 8.9.

The habituation effects are again significant.

Group A: Amplitude $T = 0$, $p < .005$
Response duration $T = 1$, $p < .025$
Group B: Amplitude $T = 0$, $p < .005$
Response duration $T = 0$, $p < .01$

Table 8.9

	Amplitude				Response duration			
	I	II	III	IV	I	II	III	IV
A	78.2	0.9	25.9	13.9	3.4	1.1	2.4	1.6
B	41.9	1.6	6.9	14.2	3.3	1.0	1.4	2.0
C	60.1	1.3	16.4	14.1	3.4	1.1	1.9	1.8

I = First response to 'traag'
II = Mean value of the last three responses to 'traag'
III = Response to 'snel'
IV = Response to 'langzaam'

A = Order 'snel', 'langzaam'
B = Order 'langzaam', 'snel'
C = Mean value of A and B

Stimulus change causes dishabituation.

Amplitude

Group A: change-over II → III : $T = 0$, $p < .005$
change-over II → IV : $T = 1$, $p < .01$
Group B: change-over II → III : $T = 1$, $p < .01$
change-over II → IV : $T = 0$, $p < .005$

Response duration

Group A: change-over II → III : $T = 0$, $p < .005$
change-over II → IV : $T = 1$, $p < .01$
Group B: change-over II → III : $T = 8.5$, n.s.
change-over II → IV : $T = 1.5$, $p < .025$

The difference between III and IV under C is not significant ($T = 83$).

Reviewing the results presented under a, b and c, we see that habituation has invariably occurred and that stimulus change causes dishabituation, particularly as regards the response amplitude. As to the nature of the new stimulus words, we must conclude that their semantic relation to the original stimulus plays no role of any significance. Irrespective of its semantic value, the second new stimulus word evokes a smaller response. This effect must be interpreted as renewed habituation after stimulus change. In all the cases of dishabituation subjects reported having perceived the stimulus change.

8.2.3

The third type of stimulus invariance explored by us concerned a number of words scaled along a certain semantic dimension.

In the previous experiment (8.2.2), the meaning variable was manipulated in the simplest possible manner, by repetition of the same stimulus word. It should also be possible, however, to use different words possessing a common characteristic, *i.e.* a more or less similar meaning. Assuming that during presentation of a sequence of such words habituation will occur, stimulation with words that have a sufficiently different semantic value from the preceding sequence, will conceivably cause dishabituation.

For an experimental test of this hypothesis we used a scale devised by Orlebeke (unpublished investigation), who had given 75 subjects a list of 80 words (adjectives) that thad to be scaled along a dimension designated as dejected – elated (9-point scale). The twenty words with the lowest scale values were now used to compose a stimulus sequence. Examples of these words are 'ellendig' (wretched), 'jammerlijk' (pitiful), 'ongelukkig' (miserable), 'treurig' (woeful), etc.

After auditory presentation of these twenty words to a group of twenty subjects, the new stimulus words 'rustig' (quiet) and 'verrukkelijk' (delightful) were given, representing the medium and highest scale values respectively. Group A received the new stimulus words in the order 'rustig – verrukkelijk', group B in the reverse order. The response data are given in tabel 8.10.

Table 8.10

	Amplitude				Response duration			
	I	II	III	IV	I	II	III	IV
A	38.9	3.0	5.0	4.2	2.9	1.5	1.0	1.4
B	37.3	0.9	1.6	2.3	2.9	0.9	1.2	0.8
C	38.1	2 0	3.3	3.3	2.9	1.2	1.1	1.1

I = First response
II = Mean value of the last three responses
III = Response to 'rustig'
IV = Response to 'verrukkelijk'

A = Order 'rustig', 'verrukkelijk'
B = Order 'verrukkelijk', 'rustig'
C = Mean value of A and B

The habituation effects are significant.

Group A: Amplitude : $T = 0$, $p < .005$
Response duration : $T = 0$, $p < .005$
Group B: Amplitude : $T = 0$, $p < .005$
Response duration : $T = 4$, $p < .10$

The dishabituation effect is not significant.

Amplitude

Group A:	Change-over: old sequence → 'rustig'	: T = 15 n.s.
	Change-over: old sequence → 'verrukkelijk'	: T = 14.5 n.s.
Group B:	Change-over: old sequence → 'rustig'	: T = 8 n.s.
	Change-over: old sequence → 'verrukkelijk'	: T = 6 $p < .10$

It seems hardly worth-wile to test the data on response duration. The results under C show that there is no difference at all between the two (new) stimulus words.

Of the 20 subjects 15 expressed the opinion that the last two words did not belong in the original sequence. All (six) cases of dishabituation were included in this number.

8.2.4

The fourth and last type of stimulus invariance was realized through the presentation of pairs of words, each exhibiting an identical semantic relation between its members. That is to say, the constant relationship within the pairs constituted the stimulus invariance. Two sequences were used.

a. In the first sequence the relationship within the pairs of words was that of contrast, as in 'schoon' (clean) – 'vuil' (dirty), 'hoog' (high) – 'laag' (low), 'arm' (poor) – 'rijk' (rich), etc, the sequence comprising twenty pairs in all. The new stimulus consisted of a pair of words of synonymous instead of contrasting meaning, *viz.* 'scherp' (sharp) – 'puntig' (pointed). The data are given in table 8.11.

Table 8.11

	I	II	III
Amplitude	28.2	2.7	0.7
Response duration	2.6	1.4	0.6

I = First response
II = Mean value of the last three responses
III = Response to new stimulus

The habituation effect is significant: Amplitude $T = 0$ $p < .005$
Response duration $T = 0$ $p < .01$

No dishabituation occurred. Only two of the ten subjects had perceived a change. In two cases a dishabituation response was given; these are the same subjects who had perceived the stimulus change.

b) In the second sequence the same mutual relationship was used in the reverse order, first similarity of meaning as in 'snel' (fast) – 'vlug' (quick), 'traag' (sluggish) – 'langzaam' (slow), etc, twenty pairs in all, and followed by the new contrasting pair 'nat' (wet) – 'droog' (dry). The response data are given in table 8.12.

Table 8.12

	I	II	III
Amplitude	23.6	1.1	0.5
Response duration	2.4	1.1	0.5

I = First response
II = Mean value of the last three responses
III = Response to the new stimulus

The habituation effect is significant: Amplitude : $T = 1$ $p < .005$
Response duration: $T = 1$ $p < .05$

Stimulus change produces no dishabituation; four of the ten subjects had perceived the change, including the two cases of dishabituation. It would appear therefore that subjects hardly if at all react to changes in this kind of semantic relationship, probably because in most cases they fail to perceive the change in interrelation.

8.3 SUMMARY

Reviewing the data on habituation and dishabituation in response to complex stimuli, we arrive at the following conclusions. Habituation occurs invariably, irrespective of the type of stimulus used. The question as to whether this habituation is actually due to the invariance of the stimuli (at any rate as seen by the experimenter) can be answered by reference to the findings on dishabituation.

As regards the number sequences, we see that the principle of the sequence does indeed play a role in dishabituation, albeit that the effect is a function of the degree of complexity.

Sound changes in sequences consisting of simple (monosyllabic) words cause little or no dishabituation. From the finding that in most cases the stimulus change is in fact perceived, we may draw the provisional conclusion that it is the words themselves rather than the vowel sounds which dominate, and that the sound change produces too slight a 'distance' between the word stimuli to cause dishabituation.

While the change-over (after habituation) from a stimulus word to a word of similar or more contrasting meaning causes dishabituation in both cases, the results do not bear out the supposition that the word of similar meaning will cause less dishabituation.

Presentation of words of a high scale value, following a sequence of words of low scale value (within the dimension 'dejected' – 'elated'), does not cause significant dishabituation (30% showed dishabituation).

Changes in the semantic relationship within pairs of words (similarity and contrast) do not give rise to dishabituation. In these cases only a few subjects had perceived the nature of the change.

From these various findings we may conclude with some reserve that the primary condition for dishabituation is that the subject should have perceived the change and that, secondly, the distance between the original and the modified stimuli should appear sufficiently large to the subject. Such factors as attention and intelligence naturally play an important part in this respect.

There is one point, however, which requires further attention. In the foregoing sections we have repeatedly seen that the subject's perception of changes in stimulation is a condition for dishabituation. But the group of subjects who perceived stimulus changes contains at least an equally large number of cases in which no dishabituation occurred as of those in which it did. The issue involved is that of the relation between cognitive processes and the OR.

Kimmel and Leckart (1969) feel that it is optimistic, to say the least, to think (as Berlyne seems to do) that cognitively mediated processes 'can be comprehended in a framework built upon observations of autonomic or cortical psychophysiological reactions'. They themselves obtained experimental evidence that in visual inspection of certain figures (18-sided randomly generated polygons) the OR (GSR component) habituated while the looking time increased systematically.

According to these authors, habituation is not due to reducedat tention. Following up this argument, it could conceivably be posited that in that case certain changes in the cognitive system need not necessarily lead to dishabituation.

Continued investigations of the type described in this chapter should primarily be directed toward determining the conditions of the stimulus situation (upon perception of stimulus changes) under which dishabituation occurs.

In this connection mention should be made of the work of Bernstein (1969), who found that about half the subjects who had clearly perceived a stimulus change showed no dishabituation. His conclusion is that 'the OR is not an automatic accompaniment to perceptible stimulus novelty'.

Bernstein has hypothesized a two-stage process in triggering an OR, in which the match-mismatch process as described by Sokolov is followed by evalution of the stimulus information. If the stimulus change is of significance to the subject, an OR will occur.

SUMMARY AND AFTERWORD

In the first part of this study a survey is given of the determinants and properties of the orientation reflex (OR), especially of the GSR component of the OR.

The determinants discussed are: novelty, change and incongruity, conflict, surprise, complexity, intensity, perceptual expectation and signal value. In addition, the relation between the OR and various memory forms as well as individual differences are dealt with.

Following out of this a survey is given of the functions of the OR, such as adjustment of the analyzers, inhibition of the ongoing behavior and the role of the OR in the conditioning process. Next, OR habituation and dishabituation are discussed. Finally, the parametric characteristics of the habituation process are reviewed as well as recent theory formation in this area, the latter focussing on Sokolov's neuronal model, including the so-called filter model.

In the second part, the author's own experimental research is set out and discussed. This research should be seen in terms of further elaboration and experimental testing of a number of hypotheses derived from Sokolov's theory of the OR. The experiments are particularly concerned with the habituation, dishabituation and signalization of the OR. One of the reasons why we have undertaken this research is that Sokolov gives no statistical analyses. This circumstance has caused several investigators to adopt a rather skeptical stance with regard to his work and that of other Russian psychophysiologists. While there have been some replications of Sokolov's experimental work, their scale has mostly been too limited. It is primarily against this background that our research should be seen.

Its central purpose has been to obtain reliable quantitative information about the nature and function of the OR. Further research on the OR is conditional on the availability of this type of data. A case in point is such applied subjects in the (clinical and non-clinical) psychology of individual differences as the ranking of individuals along psychophysiological dimensions, in which the obtained values are correlated with the psychological variables used in the diagnostic procedure. As has already become clear from the investigation described in Ch 1.2.8, such psychophysiological variables as habituation rate, spontaneous activity, response latency and amplitude, etc are used in this type of research. Little is known, however, about the interdependence of these variables.

Further information on this score is essential to permit psychophysiologically oriented research in depth in the psychology of individual differences, particularly on the problem of whether certain personality characteristics are accompanied by particular patterns of psychophysiological variables.

Quantitative knowledge of the OR parameters is also indispensable in studying the role of the OR in certain behavioral processes such as stimulus generalization, classical conditioning, skill learning, etc.

Also, there is a need for further information about the quantitative relations (interdependence) between the different response measures such as amplitude, duration and latency as well as about the trend of the prestimulus level.

The research reported in this second part primarily deals with the phenomena of OR habituation and dishabituation in response to sensory and complex stimuli. The main issues are: What parameters determine the habituation process, and under what conditions does dishabituation occur? In this context also a few more specific hypotheses have been tested, such as the supposed linear relation between the response amplitude and the log of the stimulus number in habituation, the representation of temporal stimulus properties in the neuronal model of the stimulus, and Sokolov's filter model for dishabituation. To this end, not only purely sensory but also complex stimuli (words and numbers) have been used.

In a separate chapter (7) the following additional topics have been studied: the relation between perceptual expectation and OR occurrence, the inhibitory function of the OR, and the determinants of signalization, particularly in so-called differential signalization.

Our experiments have in the main confirmed Sokolov's hypotheses, with the exception of the filter model.

In what follows the results for each of the three main subjects will be briefly summarized, and an attempt will be made to place the factual findings in a wider perspective. In all the experiments the GSR measured by the method of constant current served as OR indicator. Apart from response amplitude

($\triangle$ log C), duration and latency have also been used as response measures. All the stimuli were of an auditory nature.

1. Habituation

Stimulus repetition caused habituation in all cases, that is, irrespective of whether the stimuli were sensory or complex, with or without signal value. This habituation manifests itself in decreased response amplitude and duration and increased response latency. The habituation process proceeds more slowly if stimulus duration, stimulus intensity and/or the interstimulus interval increase. The correlations between the habituation rate (= the number of stimulations required to attain complete habituation) and the amplitude of the first response are positive but not always significant. There is a distinct tendency for habituation to proceed more slowly at higher arousal levels.

This tendency is confirmed by the positive correlation between spontaneous activity and habituation rate. The relation between response amplitude and the log stimulus number is linear.

Habituation is a very general phenomenon, which may be regarded as the most elementary form of learning, and which occurs even in planarians. Psychologically, OR habituation may be defined as a diminishing relevance of the stimulus information.

Various authors (see Lynn's survey, 1966) have pointed out that the OR and OR habituation play an important part in the process whereby conditioned responses are established. Luria (1963) has demonstrated the special significance of this fact for studies of mentally defective children. There is a clearly demonstrable relation between defective attention and poor learning on the one hand and defects of the OR mechanism and the habituation system on the other. As a result, verbal behavior regulation will develop poorly or not at all.

In Ch 2.2 mention has been made of the fact that pre-habituation of the OR to the CS seriously impedes the conditioning process. Concurrent presentation of the CS and UCS causes habituation to proceed less quickly than when these stimuli are presented separately.

Again, however, the problem is that few statistical tests are available, and further research in this area is therefore needed. In view of the fact that the Russian literature (see Lynn's survey, 1966) shows that there are all sorts of relations between the development of learning ability and the development of the OR mechanisms, this continued research should not lose sight of the developmental-psychological aspect.

It seems likely that various aspects of learning psychology would benefit from renewed investigation from the viewpoint of habituation. A case in point is the finding that massed learning tends to produce poorer learning results than spaced learning. A rapid succession of learning trials will cause the OR to the CS to habituate more quickly. If early habituation of the OR to the CS adversely affects the learning process, this might provide the explanation for the poorer learning result in massed learning. This approach to the phenomenon could be regarded as a further specification of the inhibition concept as used in the commonly accepted explanation of the difference between massed learning and spaced learning.

The learning process can also be approached from the viewpoint of individual psychophsysiological differences. Individuals are commonly divided into 'unstable' and 'stable' personalities on the basis of their spontaneous activity (non-specific GSR's). In 'stable' individuals habituation of the OR proceeds much more quickly than in 'unstable' individuals.

This had led Koepke and Pribram (1966) to postulate that individuals exhibiting more spontaneous activity ('unstable' personalities) are easier to condition (in the Pavlovian sense). They obtained confirmation for their hypothesis from data in the literature.

A final point should be made about the relation between habituation and extinction. Sokolov (1963b) points out that OR habituation shows a certain resemblance to extinction of a CR. The shape of habituation and extinction curves is the same. In both cases an inhibition process is involved. Also, disinhibition (as a result of external stimulation) and spontaneous recovery occur in both cases. The difference, however, is that the OR has not been acquired through a learning process, as the CR has, but is immediately given as an unconditioned reaction.

Apart from the above, more physiological correspondences, there would also be a psychological similarity if extinction, like habituation, could be explained in terms of diminishing relevance of the information of the conditional stimulus. This seems quite well possible since, as a result of the conditioning process, the CS has come to signal the occurrence of the UCS, which in general manifests itself in the occurrence of a conditional anticipatory response (CAR). If now the YCS is systematically omitted, the signal relevance or information value diminishes, as a result of which the CAR decreases (extinguishes).

This more cognitive interpretation of the extinction process is, in the case of autonomic conditioning, quite consistent with the phenomena of one-trial conditioning and one-trial extinction. These effects are brought about by verbal instructions. Thus, practically complete extinction of a conditioned GSR can be attained by the simple announcement that no further UCS (shock) will be presented, with simultaneous removal of the particular electrodes. In this case the announced discontinuation reduces the original information value of the CS to zero.

2. Dishabituation

The properties of the neuronal model of the stimulus, as postulated by Sokolov (1960), can best be investigated by studying the dishabituation symptoms caused by stimulus change. With one exception, the properties of the neuronal model of the stimulus as formulated by Sokolov (see Ch 3.4) have been confirmed by us. It has been proved that records of the stimulus properties duration, intensity and quality (tone frequency) become fixed in the neuronal model. A change in one of these properties causes dishabituation, which manifests itself in an increase in response amplitude and duration and frequently in a decrease in response latency.

Sokolov's theory postulates that the temporal characteristics of stimulation likewise become fixed in the model. This has been found to hold at least for stimulus duration, since our experimental evidence showed that dishabituation was indeed due to a change in stimulus duration. With regard to the interstimulus interval the picture is less clear, although we must hasten to add that in this case only limited experimental data were available. Dishabituation occurred in two of the ten cases when the interval was shortened, and in four of the ten cases when the interval was prolonged.

According to Sokolov's theory, the degree of dishabituation, regardless of the direction of stimulus change, is an increasing function of the distance between the original and the modified stimulus (the so-called filter model). No evidence whatsoever has been obtained by us in support of this hypothesis. The postulated relation was found to hold neither for the factor stimulus intensity nor for the tone frequency parameter. It must therefore be considered exteremely doubtful whether the filter model actually exists. This conclusion is in accord with the findings of Zimny and Schwabe (1965), who studied the effect of the factor tone frequency over a restricted range.

Another point concerns the generalization of intersession habituation, the so-called potentiation of habituation. Intersession habituation occurs whenever after dishabituation by another stimulus the original stimulus is again presented repeatedly. The dishabituated response, however, has a lower response strength and habituates much more quickly. Both effects are due to intersession habituation. If now, after dishabituation, not the original stimulus but the modified stimulus is repeatedly presented, there is still a certain amount of intersession habituation to be expected. This phenomenon is called generalization of intersession habituation.

The effect of intersession habituation should become apparent from a smaller response amplitude, and a longer response latency, as compared with the first response of the sequence before dishabituation. At the same time, the number of trials required to attain renewed habituation should be smaller. In general, our findings provide confirmation on this score for the stimulus properties duration, intensity and tone frequency. It should be noted that where stimulus intensity is concerned, amplitude proved to be the best response criterion for intersession habituation.

In a more exploratory experiment the occurrence of dishabituation in response to complex stimuli was studied. A problem is that the stimulus change is by no means always perceived. Number sequences, composed according to an underlying principle, cause progressive habituation on successive trials, followed by dishabituation when numbers are presented that depart from what the subject had been led to expect on the basis of the preceding stimulations. A similar finding has been obtained by Unger (1964), who used vasoconstriction (in the finger) as the dependent variable. Vowel changes and changes in the semantic relations between stimulus words in the main produced negative results. Since only a few subjects had perceived the stimulus changes, no very definite conclusions can be drawn. Further research in this area is therefore desirable.

Finally, there is the relation between dishabituation and the subject's perception of the stimulus change. From the statement of Pribram (1966) that 'subjectively, the OR is correlated with awareness, habituation with unawareness', it follows that dishabituation is correlated with awareness. Our evidence confirms this hypothesis, although there is no one-to-one correspondence. In the case of sensory stimuli, perception of the stimulus change is as a rule found to be accompanied by dishabituation. For complex stimuli this is no longer true. Sometimes only 50% of the cases in which the stimulus change was perceived exhibited dishabituation. Kimmel and Leckart (1969) have likewise shown that the relation between cognitively mediated responses and the OR is not as straightforward as has sometimes been assumed (see also: Bernstein, 1969). Further research will be needed to give us a better insight into these relations.

3. Signalization

Signalization is defined as the acquisition of signal value by a neutral stimulus. This process is brought about by classical conditioning or a verbal instruction, whether or not combined with a motor reaction. Luria and Homskaya (1964) attach great importance to signalization: 'This basic mechanism makes it possible to regulate the active state of cortical systems by means of a verbal instruction, and to bring even the vegetative components under verbal control.'

Signalization in a simple RT task was demonstrated by us from increased OR's and a much delayed habituation process. On the basis of Sokolov's (1966b) listing of the OR as a kind of 'information regulator', the hypothesis was formulated that in the signalization process the size of the OR and the habituation rate are a function of the degree of uncertainty in a sequence consisting of signal and non-signal stimuli (differential signalization). This hypothesis was confirmed.

The correlation between signalization and the degree of uncertainty is important for an analysis of partial reinforcement situations. Lovibond (1969) reports an experiment in which two stimuli (10 sec light and 1 sec buzzer) were presented in a classical conditioning paradigm with different percentages of reinforcement. This means that sometimes the light stimulus was followed by the buzzer, sometimes not. The 7 groups used received 0, 10, 20, 50, 80, 90 or 100% buzzer reinforcement.

The prediction that habituation would be slower with increasing uncertainty was fulfilled. No significant differences were found between the groups of 0 and 100%, between the groups of 10 and 90% and between those of 20 and 80% (equal degree of uncertainty). Habituation took longest for the 50% group, followed by the 20 and 80% groups, the 10 and 90% groups, and finally the 0 and 100% groups. The no-difference finding for the 0 and 100% groups indicates that uncertainty is a more important OR determinant than the amount of stimulation. Lovibond adds that it should be possible to analyze the problems associated with the acquisition and extinction effects of intermittent reinforcement in a similar manner.

4. Other results

Since all our experimental results could not be made to fit in under the three preceding heads, the other findings are listed below.

a) In our experiment on the effect of perceptual expectation on the OR, the major difficulty proved to be how to instil the perceptual expectation patterns. Only in the simplest case was it possible to demonstrate that the incongruity between the induced expectation and the actual stimulation was OR-evocative. In the absence of continued research, very little can be said on this subject with any certainty.

b) The hypothesis that a change in the tone frequency of an auditory stimulus in an RT task will evoke a OR accompanied by inhibition of the ongoing behavior was confirmed. This finding is in accord with the views of Anokhin (1965).

c) Of the various stimulus properties only stimulus intensity was found to determine OR strength. A positive linear relation was observed to exist between stimulus intensity and response amplitude. OR latency was found to decrease with increasing stimulus intensity.

d) Response amplitude and response duration were found to exhibit positive, low correlations, which were mostly not significant. An exception was observed for the group within which the stimulus intensity was varied ($r = .49$ $p < .005$). The conclusion was drawn that the form of the response wave is not entirely dependent on the response amplitude.
Negative correlations were observed to exist between amplitude and latency. This indicates that stronger responses have shorter latencies.

e) No correlation was found to exist between the amplitude of the first response and the pre-stimulus level. A slightly less favorable picture obtains for the second response. In consequence, $\triangle$ log C cannot be considered a completely base-independent measure.

f) In view of the large individual differences in responsivity, experimental subjects should, whenever possible, be used as their own controls.

REFERENCES

ALLEN, C.K., HILL, F.A., WICKENS, D.D. (1963), 'The orienting reflex as a function of the interstimulus interval of compound stimuli.' *J. Exp. Psychol.* 65, 309–316.

ANOKHIN, P.K. (1965), 'The role of the orienting-exploratory reaction in the formation of the conditioned reflex.' In: *Russian monographs on brain and behavior nr. 3. Orienting reflex and exploratory behavior.* Ed. American Institute of Biological Sciences, Washington.

ASAFOV, B.D. (1965), 'Change in the dynamics of autonomic components of the orienting reflex with the employment of sound stimuli of progressively increasing intensity.' In: *Russian monographs on brain and behavior nr. 3. Orienting reflex and exploratory behavior.* Ed. American Institute of Biological Sciences, Washington.

BERLYNE, D.E. (1960), *Conflict, arousal and curiosity.* Mc Graw-Hill, New York.

BERLYNE, D.E. (1961), 'Conflict and the orientation reaction.' *J. Exp. Psychol.* 62. 476–483.

BERLYNE, D.E., CRAW, M.A., SALAPATEK, P.H., LEWIS, J.L. (1963), 'Novelty, complexity, incongruity, extrinsic motivation, and the GSR.' *J. Exp. Psychol.* 66, 560–567.

BERLYNE, D.E., BOSRA, D.M. (1968), 'Uncertainty and the orientation reaction.' *Percep. and Psychophys.*, 3, 77–79.

BERNSTEIN, A.S. (1968), 'The orienting response and direction of stimulus change.' *Psychon. Sci.* 12, 127–128.

BERNSTEIN, A.S. (1969), 'To what does the orienting response respond.' *Psychophysiol.* 6, 338–350.

BONVALLET, M., DELL, P., HIEBEL, G. (1954), 'Tonus sympathique et activité électrique corticale.' *EEG Clin. Neurophysiol.* 6, 119–144.

BRUNER, J.S. (1951) 'Personality dynamics and the process of perceiving.' In: R.R. Blake and G.V. Ramsey. *Perception. An approach to personality.* Ronald, New York.

CHATTERJEE, B.B., ERIKSEN, C.W. (1960), 'Conditioning and generalization of GSR as a function of awareness.' *J. Abn. Soc. Psychol.* 60, 396–403.

CHATTERJEE, B.B., ERIKSEN, C.W. (1962), 'Cognitive factors in heart rate conditioning.' *J. Exp. Psychol.* 64, 272–279.

COOMBS, C.H. (1938), 'Adaptation of the galvanic response to auditory stimuli.' *J. Exp. Psychol.* 22, 244–268.

COSTELL, R.M., LEIDERMANN, P.H. (1968), 'Psychophysiological concomitants of social stress: the effects of conformity pressure.' *Psychosom. Med.* 30, 298–310.

DARROW, C.W. (1937), 'The equation of the galvanic skin reflex curve: I. The dynamics of reaction in relation to excitation background.' *J. Gen. Psychol.* 16, 285–309.

DAVIS, R.C. (1934), 'Modification of the galvanic reflex by daily repetition of a stimulus.' *J. Exp. Psychol.* 17, 504–535.

DAVIS, R.C., BUCHWALD, A.M., FRANKMANN, R.W. (1955), 'Autonomic and muscular responses and their relation to simple stimuli.' *Psychol. Monogr.* 69, no. 405.

DEESE, J. (1958), *The psychology of learning.* Mc. Graw-Hill, New York.

DELL, P. (1963), 'Reticular homeostasis and critical reactivity.' In: G. Moruzzi a.o. *Progress in Brain Research*, Vol. I. Elsevier, Amsterdam.

DYKMAN, R.A., REESE, W.G., GALBRECHT, C.R., THOMASSON, P.J. (1959), 'Psychophysiological reactions to novel stimuli: measurement, adaptation and relationship of psychological and physiological variables in the normal human.' *Ann. New Y. Acad. Sci.* 79, 43–107.

DYKMAN, R.A. (1967), 'On the nature of classical conditioning.' In: C.C. Brown: *Methods in psychophysiology*, ch. 11. The Williams and Wilkins Company, Baltimore.

EDELBERG R. (1967) 'Electrical properties of the skin.' In: C.C. Brown: *Psychophysiological methods*, Ch 1. The Williams and Wilkins Company, Baltimore.

EDWARDS, A.L. (1960), *Experimental design in psychological research.* Holt, Rinehart and Winston, New York.

FRIED, R., KORN, S.J., Welch, L. (1966), 'Effect of change in sequential stimuli on GSR adaptation.' *J. Exp. Psychol.* 72, 325–327.

FRIED, R., WELCH, L., FRIEDMANN, M., GLUCK S. (1967), 'Is no stimulus a stimulus?' *J. Exp. Psychol.* 73, 145–146.

FUREDY, J.J. (1968), 'Novelty and the measurement of the GSR.' *J. Exp. Psychol.* 76, 501–503.

FUREDY, J.J. (1969) 'Some uses and abuses of electrodermal measures.' *Psychon. Sci.*, 15, 98–99.

GALBRECHT, C.R., DYKMAN, R.A., REESE, W.G., SUZUKI, T. (1965), 'Intrasession adaptation and intersession extinction of the components of the orienting response.' *J. Exp. Psychol.* 70, 585–597.

GEER, J.H. (1966), 'Effect of interstimulus intervals and rest-period length upon habituation of the orienting response.' *J. Exp. Psychol.* 72, 617–619.

GEER, J.H. (1967), 'Some basic parameters of the orienting response.' In: I. Ruttkay-Nedecky a.o.: *Mechanism of orienting reaction in man.* Publishing House of Slovak Academy of Sciences, Bratislava.

GORMEZANO, I. (1966), 'Classical conditioning.' In: J.B. Sidowski: *Experimental methods and instrumentation in psychology.* Mc Graw-Hill, New York.

GRANIT, R. (1955), *Receptors and sensory perception.* Yale University Press, New Haven.

GREENFIELD, N.S., ALEXANDER, A.A., ROESSLER, R. (1963), 'Ego strength and physiological responsivity II.' *Arch. Gen. Psychiatr.* 9, 129–141.

GRINGS, W.W. (1960), 'Preparatory set variables related to conditioning of autonomic responses.' *Psychol. Rev.* 67, 243–252.

HARRIS, D.J. (1943), 'Habituatory response decrement in the intact organism.' *Psychol. Bull.* 40, 385–422.

HAYES, R., BRONSAFT, A., BLOCH, M., WELCH, L., (1964), 'Intraseries primacy and the orienting reflex of the GSR.' *J. Psychol.* 58, 107–113.

HAYS, W.L. (1963), *Statistics for psychologists*. Holt, Rinehart and Winston, New York.

HIND, J.E., ROSE, J.E., DAVIES, P.W., WOOLSEY, C.N., BENJAMIN, R.M., WELKER, W.I., THOMPSON, R.F. (1961), 'Unit activity in the auditory cortex.' In: G.L, Rasmussen and W.F. Windle: *Neural mechanisms of the auditory and vestibular systems*. Charles C. Thomas, Springfield Ill.

HOVLAND, C.I., RIESSEN, S.H. (1940), 'Magnitude of galvanic and vasomotor response as a function of stimulus intensity.' *J. Gen. Psychol.* 23, 103–121.

JOHNSON, L.C. (1963), 'Some attributes of spontaneous autonomic activity.' *J. Comp. Physiol. Psychol.* 56, 415–422.

KAPLAN, H.B., BURCH, N.R., BLOOM, S.W. (1965), 'Physiological covariation and sociometric relationships in small peer groups.' In: P.H. Leiderman and D. Shapiro: *Psychobiological approaches to social behavior*. Tavistock, London.

KIMMEL, H.D. (1960), 'The relationship between direction and amount of stimulus change and amount of perceptual disparity response.' *J. Exp. Psychol.* 59, 68–72.

KIMMEL, H.D., KIMMEL, E. (1965), 'Sex differences in adaptation of the GSR under repeated applications of a visual stimulus.' *J. Exp. Psychol.* 70, 536–537.

KIMMEL, H.D. and LECKART, B.T. (1969), 'Paired comparison scaling of reaction potential from simultaneous measurements of GSR and looking time.' *Percep. Psychophys.*, 5, 294–296.

KOEPKE, J.E., PRIBRAM, K.H. (1966), 'Habituation of GSR as a function of stimulus duration and spontaneous activity.' *J. Comp. Physiol.* 61, 442–448.

KOEPKE, J.E., PRIBRAM, K.H. (1967), 'Habituation of the vasoconstriction response as a function of stimulus duration and anxiety.' *J. Comp. Physiol. Psychol.* 64, 502–504.

KORN, J.H., MOYER, K.E. (1968), 'Effects of set and sex on the electrodermal orienting response.' *Psychophysiol.* 4, 453–459.

LADER, M.H. and WING, L. (1964), 'Habituation of the psycho-galvanic reflex in patients with anxiety states and in normal subjects.' *J. Neurol. Neurosurg. Psychiat.* 27, 210–218.

LEAVY, A., GEER, J.H. (1967), 'The effect of low levels of stimulus intensity upon the orienting response.' *Psychon. Sci.* 9, 105–106.

LOVIBOND, S.H. (1969), 'Habituation of the orienting response to multiple stimulus sequences.' *Psychophysiol.* 5, 435–439.

LUBORSKY, L. (1967), 'Individual differences in cognitive style as a determinant of vasoconstrictive orienting responses. In: I. Ruttkay-Nedecky a.o.: *Mechanisms of orienting reaction in man*, 73–81. Publishing House of Slovak Academy of Sciences, Bratislava.

LURIA, A.R., VINOGRADOVA, O.S. (1959), 'An objective investigation of the dynamics of semantic systems.' *Brit. J. Psychol.* 50, 89–105.

LURIA, A.R. (1963), *The mentally retarded child*. Pergamon Press, Oxford.

LURIA, A.R. and HOMSKAYA, E.D. (1964), 'Disturbance in the regulative role of speech with frontal lobe lesions.' In: J.M. Warren and K. Akert (eds.): *The frontal granular cortex and behavior*, 353–371. Mc. Graw-Hill, New York.

LYNN, R. (1966), *Attention, arousal and the orientation reaction*. Pergamon Press, Oxford·

MONTAGU, J.D., COLES, E.M. (1966) 'Mechanism and measurement of the galvanic skin response.' *Psychol. Bull.* 65, 261.279.

NOWLIN, J.B., Eisdorfer, C., BOGDONOFF, M.D., NICHOLS, C.R. (1968), 'Physiologic response to active and passive participation in a two-person interaction.' *Psychosom. Med.* 30, 87–94.

OLST, E.H. VAN, ORLEBEKE, J.F., FOKKEMA, S.D. (1966), 'The role of the orienting reflex in the generalization of a conditioned GSR (II).' In: *Orienting reflex, alertness and attention*. Proceedings of the XVIIIth International Congress of Psychology, Symposium 5.

OLST, E.H. VAN, HAM, F. VAN DER (1967), 'Enkele problemen bij de bepaling van de electro-dermale response.' *Nederl. Tijdschr. Psychol.* 22, 301–313.

OLST, E.H. VAN, ORLEBEKE, J.F. (1967), 'An analysis of the concept of arousal.' *Ned. Tijdschr. Psychol.* 22, 583–603.

ORLEBEKE, J.F., OLST, E.H. VAN (1968), 'Learning and performance as a function of CS intensity in a delayed GSR conditioning situation.' *J. Exp. Psychol.* 77, 483–487.

OSWALD, I. (1962), *Sleeping and waking*. Elsevier, Amsterdam.

PAVLOV, I.P. (1927), *Conditioned reflexes*. Clarendon Press, Oxford.

PORTER, J.M. (1938), 'Adaptation of the galvanic skin response.' *J. Exp. Psychol.* 23, 553–557.

PRIBRAM, K.H. (1963), 'Reinforcement revisited: a structural view.' In: M.R. Jones (ed.): *Nebraska symposium on motivation*. University of Nebraska Press.

PRIBRAM, K.H. (1966), 'Some dimensions of remembering: steps toward a neuropsychological model of memory.' In: J. Gaito (ed.): *Macromolecules and behavior*, 166–173. Academic Press, New York.

PROKASY, W.F., HALL, J.F. (1963), 'Primary stimulus generalization.' *Psychol. Rev.* 70, 310–322.

RACKMAN, S. (1960), 'Reliability of galvanic response measures.' *Psychol. Rep.* 6, 326.

ROBINSON, D.W., DADSON, R.S. (1957), 'Threshold of hearing and equal-loudness relations for pure tones and the loudness function.' *J. Acoust. Soc. Amer.* 29, 1284–1288.

ROESSLER, R., ALEXANDER, A.A., GREENFIELD, N.S. (1963), 'Ego strength and physiological rèsponsivity I.' *Arch. Gen. Psychiatr.* 8, 142–154.

ROSENHAN, D., MESSICK, S. (1966), 'Affect and expectation.' *J. Pers. Soc. Psychol.* 3, 38–44.

SHAPIRO, D., LEIDERMAN, P.H. (1965), 'Acts and activation: A psychophysiological study of social interaction.' In: P.H. Leiderman and D. Shapiro: *Psychobiological approaches to social behavior*. Tavistock, London.

SHARPLESS, S., JASPER, H. (1956), 'Habituation of the arousal reaction.' *Brain*, 79, 655–681.

SHEAN, G.D. (1968), 'Vasomotor conditioning and awareness.' *Psychophysiol.* 5, 22–30.

SIEGEL, S. (1956), *Nonparametric statistics for the behavioral sciences*. Mc Graw-Hill, New York.

SOKOLOV, E.N. (1960), 'Neuronal models and the orienting reflex.' In: M.A.B. Brazier, *The central nervous system and behavior*. Third conference, Josiah Macy Jr. Foundation, Boston.

SOKOLOV, E.N. (1963a), 'Higher nervous functions: the orienting reflex.' *Ann. Rev. Physiol.*

SOKOLOV, E.N. (1963b), *Perception and the conditioned reflex*. Pergamon Press, Oxford.

SOKOLOV, E.N. (1966a) 'Neuronal mechanisms of the orienting reflex.' In: *Orienting reflex, alterness, and attention*. Proceedings of the XVIIIth International Congress of Psychology. Symposium 5.

SOKOLOV, E.N. (1966b), 'Orienting reflex as information regulator.' In: A. Leontyev a.o.: *Psychological research in the USSR*. Progress Publishers, Moscow.

SOKOLOV, E.N. (1967) 'Die reflektorischen Grundlagen der Wahrnemung.' In: H. Hiebsch: '*Ergebnisse der sowjetischen Psychologie*'. Akademie-Verlag, Berlin.

SOLLEY, C.M., MURPHY, G. (1960), *Development of the perceptual world*. Basic Books, New York.

STEIN L. (1966), 'Habituation and stimulus novelty: A model based on classical conditioning.' *Psychol. Rev.* 73, 352–356.

STERN, J.A. (1964), 'Toward a definition of psychophysiology.' *Psychophysiol.* 1, 90–92.

STERN, J.A. (1968), 'Toward a developmental psychophysiology: My look into the crystal ball.' *Psychophysiol.* 4 403–420.

STERNBACH R.A. (1964), 'The effects of instructional sets on autonomic responsivity.' *Psychophysiol.* 1, 67–72.

THOMAS, D.E., KORR, I.M. (1957), 'Relationship between sweat gland activity and electrical resistance of the skin.' *J. Appl. Physiol.* 10, 505–510.

THOMPSON, R.F. (1965).'The neural basis of stimulus generalization'. In: D.I. Mostofsky: *Stimulus generalization*. Stanford University Press, Standford.

THOMPSON, R.F., SPENCER, W.A. (1966), 'Habituation: A model phenomenon for the study of neuronal substrates of behavior.' *Psychol. Rev.* 73, 16–43.

THOMPSON, R.F. (1967), *Foundations of physiological psychology*. Harper and Row, New York.

THORPE W.H. (1956) *Learning and instinct in animals*. Methuen, London.

UNGER, S.M. (1964), 'Habituation of the vasoconstrictive orienting reaction.' *J. Exp. Psychol.* 67, 11–18.

UNO, T., GRINGS, W.W. (1965), 'Autonomic components of orienting behavior.' *Psychophysiol.* 1, 311–321.

VINOGRADOVA, C.S. (1966), 'Investigation of habituation in single neurons of different brain structures with special reference to the hippocampus.' In: *Orienting reflex, alertness and attention.* Proceedings of the XVIIIth International Congress of Psychology, symposium 5. Moscow.

VORONIN, L.G., SOKOLOV, E.N. (1960), 'Cortical mechanisms of the orienting reflex and its relation to the conditioned reflex.' *E.E.G. Clin. Neurophysiol.* suppl. 13.

WEINER, B., FELDMAN, P., (1967), 'Information processing related to stimulus novelty and complexity in a signal detection paradigm.' *Brit. J. Psychol.* 58, 69–75.

WICKENS, D.D., WICKENS, C.D. (1942), 'Factors related to pseudoconditioning.' *J. Exp. Psychol.* 31, 518–526.

WILLIAMS, J.A. (1963), 'Novelty, GSR, and stimulus generalization.' *Canad. J. Psychol.* 17, 52–61.

WOLFENSBERGER, W., O'CONNOR, N. (1967), 'Relative effectiveness of galvanic skin response latency, amplitude and duration scores as measures of arousal and habituation in normal and retarded adults.' *Psychophysiol.* 3, 345–350.

ZIMNY, G.H., Schwabe, L.W. (1965), 'Stimulus change and habituation of the orienting response.' *Psychophysiol.* 2, 103–115.

ZIMNY, G.H., KIENSTRA, R.A. (1967), 'Orienting and defensive responses to electric shock.' *Psychophysiol.* 3, 351–362.

Bei Fragen zur Produktsicherheit wenden Sie sich bitte an:
If you have any questions regarding product safety,
please contact:

Walter de Gruyter GmbH
Genthiner Straße 13
10785 Berlin
productsafety@degruyterbrill.com